# THIS BOOK BELONGS TO

# BODY PROGRESS TRACKER
## MONTH/YEAR

### WAIST

Week 1: ___________

Week 2: ___________

Week 3: ___________

Week 4: ___________

### ARMS

Week 1: ___________

Week 2: ___________

Week 3: ___________

Week 4: ___________

### THIGHS

Week 1: ___________

Week 2: ___________

Week 3: ___________

Week 4: ___________

### HIPS

Week 1: ___________

Week 2: ___________

Week 3: ___________

Week 4: ___________

| Goal Tracker | Week 1: | Week 2: | Week 3: | Week 4: |
| --- | --- | --- | --- | --- |
| DATE | | | | |
| ARMS | | | | |
| WAIST | | | | |
| HIPS | | | | |
| THIGHS | | | | |
| WEIGHT | | | | |

# BODY MEASUREMENTS TRACKER

## MONTH/YEAR

| BEFORE | AFTER |
| --- | --- |
| DATE | DATE |
| CHEST | CHEST |
| LEFT ARM | LEFT ARM |
| RIGHT ARM | RIGHT ARM |
| WAIST | WAIST |
| HIPS | HIPS |
| LEFT THIGH | LEFT THIGH |
| RIGHT THIGH | RIGHT THIGH |
| LEFT CALF | LEFT CALF |
| RIGHT CALF | RIGHT CALF |
| WEIGHT | WEIGHT |

NOTES

# BODY GOALS

MONTH/YEAR . . . . . . . . . . .

### THIS MONTH GOALS

### WEEKLY PRIORITIES

W1
W2
W3
W4

### OTHER TASKS

### MONTHLY AFFIRMATION

### REVIEW OF THE MONTH

### NOTES

# *WATER CHALLENGE*

MONTH/YEAR.................

| DAYS | WATER | DAYS | WATER |
|------|-------|------|-------|
| 01 | | 16 | |
| 02 | | 17 | |
| 03 | | 18 | |
| 04 | | 19 | |
| 05 | | 20 | |
| 06 | | 21 | |
| 07 | | 22 | |
| 08 | | 23 | |
| 09 | | 24 | |
| 10 | | 25 | |
| 11 | | 26 | |
| 12 | | 27 | |
| 13 | | 28 | |
| 14 | | 29 | |
| 15 | | 30 | |

# BODY PROGRESS TRACKER

## MONTH/YEAR

### WAIST

Week 1: _______________

Week 2: _______________

Week 3: _______________

Week 4: _______________

### ARMS

Week 1: _______________

Week 2: _______________

Week 3: _______________

Week 4: _______________

### THIGHS

Week 1: _______________

Week 2: _______________

Week 3: _______________

Week 4: _______________

### HIPS

Week 1: _______________

Week 2: _______________

Week 3: _______________

Week 4: _______________

| Goal Tracker | Week 1: | Week 2: | Week 3: | Week 4: |
|---|---|---|---|---|
| DATE | | | | |
| ARMS | | | | |
| WAIST | | | | |
| HIPS | | | | |
| THIGHS | | | | |
| WEIGHT | | | | |

# BODY MEASUREMENTS TRACKER

## MONTH/YEAR

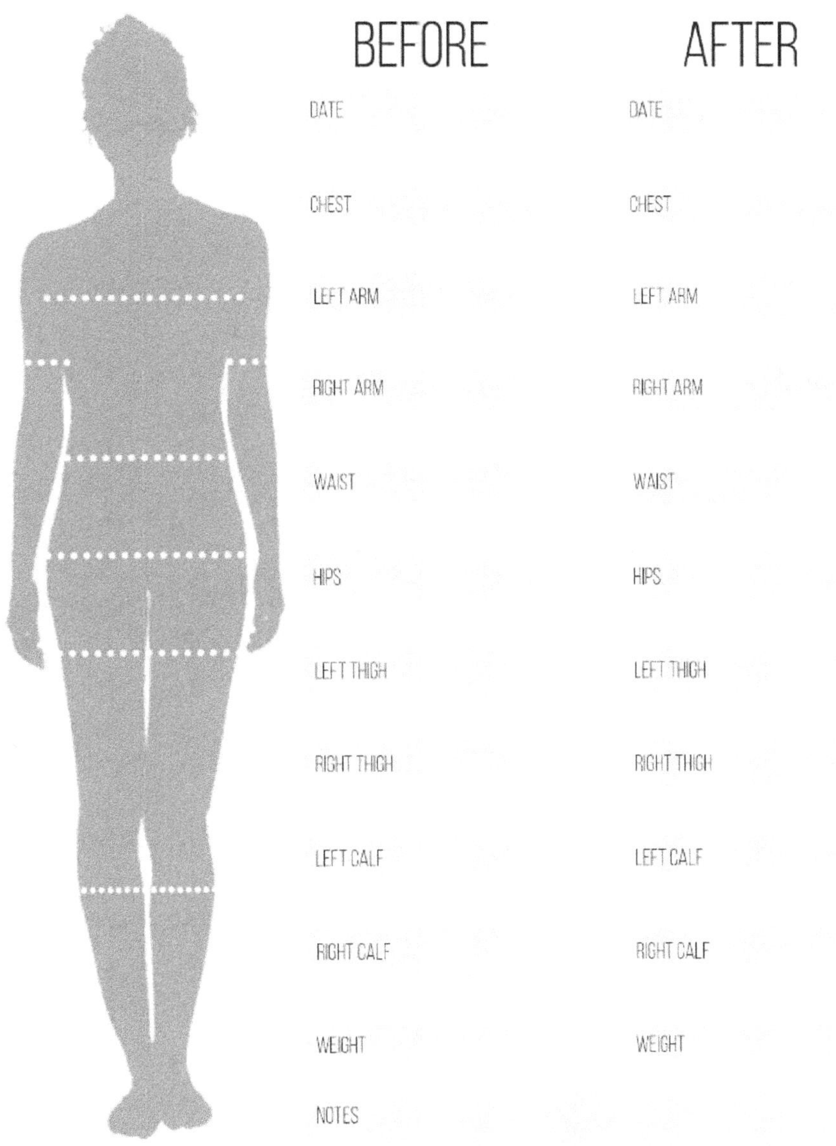

# BODY GOALS

MONTH/YEAR . . . . . . . . . . . .

## THIS MONTH
## GOALS

### WEEKLY PRIORITIES

W1

W2

W3

W4

### OTHER TASKS

### MONTHLY AFFIRMATION

### REVIEW OF THE MONTH

### NOTES

# WATER CHALLENGE

MONTH/YEAR.................

| DAYS | WATER | DAYS | WATER |
|------|-------|------|-------|
| 01 | ☐ ☐ ☐ ☐ ☐ ☐ ☐ ☐ | 16 | ☐ ☐ ☐ ☐ ☐ ☐ ☐ ☐ |
| 02 | ☐ ☐ ☐ ☐ ☐ ☐ ☐ ☐ | 17 | ☐ ☐ ☐ ☐ ☐ ☐ ☐ ☐ |
| 03 | ☐ ☐ ☐ ☐ ☐ ☐ ☐ ☐ | 18 | ☐ ☐ ☐ ☐ ☐ ☐ ☐ ☐ |
| 04 | ☐ ☐ ☐ ☐ ☐ ☐ ☐ ☐ | 19 | ☐ ☐ ☐ ☐ ☐ ☐ ☐ ☐ |
| 05 | ☐ ☐ ☐ ☐ ☐ ☐ ☐ ☐ | 20 | ☐ ☐ ☐ ☐ ☐ ☐ ☐ ☐ |
| 06 | ☐ ☐ ☐ ☐ ☐ ☐ ☐ ☐ | 21 | ☐ ☐ ☐ ☐ ☐ ☐ ☐ ☐ |
| 07 | ☐ ☐ ☐ ☐ ☐ ☐ ☐ ☐ | 22 | ☐ ☐ ☐ ☐ ☐ ☐ ☐ ☐ |
| 08 | ☐ ☐ ☐ ☐ ☐ ☐ ☐ ☐ | 23 | ☐ ☐ ☐ ☐ ☐ ☐ ☐ ☐ |
| 09 | ☐ ☐ ☐ ☐ ☐ ☐ ☐ ☐ | 24 | ☐ ☐ ☐ ☐ ☐ ☐ ☐ ☐ |
| 10 | ☐ ☐ ☐ ☐ ☐ ☐ ☐ ☐ | 25 | ☐ ☐ ☐ ☐ ☐ ☐ ☐ ☐ |
| 11 | ☐ ☐ ☐ ☐ ☐ ☐ ☐ ☐ | 26 | ☐ ☐ ☐ ☐ ☐ ☐ ☐ ☐ |
| 12 | ☐ ☐ ☐ ☐ ☐ ☐ ☐ ☐ | 27 | ☐ ☐ ☐ ☐ ☐ ☐ ☐ ☐ |
| 13 | ☐ ☐ ☐ ☐ ☐ ☐ ☐ ☐ | 28 | ☐ ☐ ☐ ☐ ☐ ☐ ☐ ☐ |
| 14 | ☐ ☐ ☐ ☐ ☐ ☐ ☐ ☐ | 29 | ☐ ☐ ☐ ☐ ☐ ☐ ☐ ☐ |
| 15 | ☐ ☐ ☐ ☐ ☐ ☐ ☐ ☐ | 30 | ☐ ☐ ☐ ☐ ☐ ☐ ☐ ☐ |

# BODY PROGRESS TRACKER

## MONTH/YEAR

### WAIST

Week 1: _____________

Week 2: _____________

Week 3: _____________

Week 4: _____________

### ARMS

Week 1: _____________

Week 2: _____________

Week 3: _____________

Week 4: _____________

### THIGHS

Week 1: _____________

Week 2: _____________

Week 3: _____________

Week 4: _____________

### HIPS

Week 1: _____________

Week 2: _____________

Week 3: _____________

Week 4: _____________

| Goal Tracker | Week 1: | Week 2: | Week 3: | Week 4: |
|---|---|---|---|---|
| DATE | | | | |
| ARMS | | | | |
| WAIST | | | | |
| HIPS | | | | |
| THIGHS | | | | |
| WEIGHT | | | | |

# BODY MEASUREMENTS TRACKER
## MONTH/YEAR

| | BEFORE | AFTER |
|---|---|---|
| DATE | | |
| CHEST | | |
| LEFT ARM | | |
| RIGHT ARM | | |
| WAIST | | |
| HIPS | | |
| LEFT THIGH | | |
| RIGHT THIGH | | |
| LEFT CALF | | |
| RIGHT CALF | | |
| WEIGHT | | |
| NOTES | | |

# BODY GOALS

MONTH/YEAR . . . . . . . . . . .

### THIS MONTH GOALS

### WEEKLY PRIORITIES

W1
W2
W3
W4

### OTHER TASKS

### MONTHLY AFFIRMATION

### REVIEW OF THE MONTH

### NOTES

# WATER CHALLENGE

MONTH/YEAR.................

| DAYS | WATER | DAYS | WATER |
|------|-------|------|-------|
| 01 | ☐ ☐ ☐ ☐ ☐ ☐ ☐ ☐ | 16 | ☐ ☐ ☐ ☐ ☐ ☐ ☐ ☐ |
| 02 | ☐ ☐ ☐ ☐ ☐ ☐ ☐ ☐ | 17 | ☐ ☐ ☐ ☐ ☐ ☐ ☐ ☐ |
| 03 | ☐ ☐ ☐ ☐ ☐ ☐ ☐ ☐ | 18 | ☐ ☐ ☐ ☐ ☐ ☐ ☐ ☐ |
| 04 | ☐ ☐ ☐ ☐ ☐ ☐ ☐ ☐ | 19 | ☐ ☐ ☐ ☐ ☐ ☐ ☐ ☐ |
| 05 | ☐ ☐ ☐ ☐ ☐ ☐ ☐ ☐ | 20 | ☐ ☐ ☐ ☐ ☐ ☐ ☐ ☐ |
| 06 | ☐ ☐ ☐ ☐ ☐ ☐ ☐ ☐ | 21 | ☐ ☐ ☐ ☐ ☐ ☐ ☐ ☐ |
| 07 | ☐ ☐ ☐ ☐ ☐ ☐ ☐ ☐ | 22 | ☐ ☐ ☐ ☐ ☐ ☐ ☐ ☐ |
| 08 | ☐ ☐ ☐ ☐ ☐ ☐ ☐ ☐ | 23 | ☐ ☐ ☐ ☐ ☐ ☐ ☐ ☐ |
| 09 | ☐ ☐ ☐ ☐ ☐ ☐ ☐ ☐ | 24 | ☐ ☐ ☐ ☐ ☐ ☐ ☐ ☐ |
| 10 | ☐ ☐ ☐ ☐ ☐ ☐ ☐ ☐ | 25 | ☐ ☐ ☐ ☐ ☐ ☐ ☐ ☐ |
| 11 | ☐ ☐ ☐ ☐ ☐ ☐ ☐ ☐ | 26 | ☐ ☐ ☐ ☐ ☐ ☐ ☐ ☐ |
| 12 | ☐ ☐ ☐ ☐ ☐ ☐ ☐ ☐ | 27 | ☐ ☐ ☐ ☐ ☐ ☐ ☐ ☐ |
| 13 | ☐ ☐ ☐ ☐ ☐ ☐ ☐ ☐ | 28 | ☐ ☐ ☐ ☐ ☐ ☐ ☐ ☐ |
| 14 | ☐ ☐ ☐ ☐ ☐ ☐ ☐ ☐ | 29 | ☐ ☐ ☐ ☐ ☐ ☐ ☐ ☐ |
| 15 | ☐ ☐ ☐ ☐ ☐ ☐ ☐ ☐ | 30 | ☐ ☐ ☐ ☐ ☐ ☐ ☐ ☐ |

# BODY PROGRESS TRACKER

## MONTH/YEAR

### WAIST

Week 1: __________
Week 2: __________
Week 3: __________
Week 4: __________

### ARMS

Week 1: __________
Week 2: __________
Week 3: __________
Week 4: __________

### THIGHS

Week 1: __________
Week 2: __________
Week 3: __________
Week 4: __________

### HIPS

Week 1: __________
Week 2: __________
Week 3: __________
Week 4: __________

| Goal Tracker | Week 1: | Week 2: | Week 3: | Week 4: |
|---|---|---|---|---|
| DATE | | | | |
| ARMS | | | | |
| WAIST | | | | |
| HIPS | | | | |
| THIGHS | | | | |
| WEIGHT | | | | |

# BODY MEASUREMENTS TRACKER
## MONTH/YEAR

| | BEFORE | AFTER |
|---|---|---|
| DATE | | |
| CHEST | | |
| LEFT ARM | | |
| RIGHT ARM | | |
| WAIST | | |
| HIPS | | |
| LEFT THIGH | | |
| RIGHT THIGH | | |
| LEFT CALF | | |
| RIGHT CALF | | |
| WEIGHT | | |
| NOTES | | |

# BODY GOALS

MONTH/YEAR . . . . . . . . . . .

## THIS MONTH GOALS

## WEEKLY PRIORITIES

*W1*

*W2*

*W3*

*W4*

## OTHER TASKS

## MONTHLY AFFIRMATION

## REVIEW OF THE MONTH

## NOTES

# WATER CHALLENGE

MONTH/YEAR.................

| DAYS | WATER | DAYS | WATER |
|------|-------|------|-------|
| 01 |  | 16 |  |
| 02 |  | 17 |  |
| 03 |  | 18 |  |
| 04 |  | 19 |  |
| 05 |  | 20 |  |
| 06 |  | 21 |  |
| 07 |  | 22 |  |
| 08 |  | 23 |  |
| 09 |  | 24 |  |
| 10 |  | 25 |  |
| 11 |  | 26 |  |
| 12 |  | 27 |  |
| 13 |  | 28 |  |
| 14 |  | 29 |  |
| 15 |  | 30 |  |

# BODY PROGRESS TRACKER

## MONTH/YEAR

### WAIST

Week 1: _______________

Week 2: _______________

Week 3: _______________

Week 4: _______________

### ARMS

Week 1: _______________

Week 2: _______________

Week 3: _______________

Week 4: _______________

### THIGHS

Week 1: _______________

Week 2: _______________

Week 3: _______________

Week 4: _______________

### HIPS

Week 1: _______________

Week 2: _______________

Week 3: _______________

Week 4: _______________

| Goal Tracker | Week 1: | Week 2: | Week 3: | Week 4: |
|---|---|---|---|---|
| DATE | | | | |
| ARMS | | | | |
| WAIST | | | | |
| HIPS | | | | |
| THIGHS | | | | |
| WEIGHT | | | | |

# BODY MEASUREMENTS TRACKER

## MONTH/YEAR

| BEFORE | AFTER |
|---|---|
| DATE | DATE |
| CHEST | CHEST |
| LEFT ARM | LEFT ARM |
| RIGHT ARM | RIGHT ARM |
| WAIST | WAIST |
| HIPS | HIPS |
| LEFT THIGH | LEFT THIGH |
| RIGHT THIGH | RIGHT THIGH |
| LEFT CALF | LEFT CALF |
| RIGHT CALF | RIGHT CALF |
| WEIGHT | WEIGHT |
| NOTES | |

# BODY GOALS

MONTH/YEAR . . . . . . . . . . .

## THIS MONTH
## GOALS

### WEEKLY PRIORITIES

*W1*

*W2*

*W3*

*W4*

### OTHER TASKS

### MONTHLY AFFIRMATION

### REVIEW OF THE MONTH

### NOTES

# *WATER CHALLENGE*

MONTH/YEAR................

| DAYS | WATER | DAYS | WATER |
|------|-------|------|-------|
| 01 | | 16 | |
| 02 | | 17 | |
| 03 | | 18 | |
| 04 | | 19 | |
| 05 | | 20 | |
| 06 | | 21 | |
| 07 | | 22 | |
| 08 | | 23 | |
| 09 | | 24 | |
| 10 | | 25 | |
| 11 | | 26 | |
| 12 | | 27 | |
| 13 | | 28 | |
| 14 | | 29 | |
| 15 | | 30 | |

# BODY PROGRESS TRACKER

## MONTH/YEAR

### WAIST

Week 1: _______________

Week 2: _______________

Week 3: _______________

Week 4: _______________

### ARMS

Week 1: _______________

Week 2: _______________

Week 3: _______________

Week 4: _______________

### THIGHS

Week 1: _______________

Week 2: _______________

Week 3: _______________

Week 4: _______________

### HIPS

Week 1: _______________

Week 2: _______________

Week 3: _______________

Week 4: _______________

| Goal Tracker | Week 1: | Week 2: | Week 3: | Week 4: |
|---|---|---|---|---|
| DATE | | | | |
| ARMS | | | | |
| WAIST | | | | |
| HIPS | | | | |
| THIGHS | | | | |
| WEIGHT | | | | |

# BODY MEASUREMENTS TRACKER

## MONTH/YEAR

| BEFORE | AFTER |
| --- | --- |
| DATE | DATE |
| CHEST | CHEST |
| LEFT ARM | LEFT ARM |
| RIGHT ARM | RIGHT ARM |
| WAIST | WAIST |
| HIPS | HIPS |
| LEFT THIGH | LEFT THIGH |
| RIGHT THIGH | RIGHT THIGH |
| LEFT CALF | LEFT CALF |
| RIGHT CALF | RIGHT CALF |
| WEIGHT | WEIGHT |

NOTES

# BODY GOALS

MONTH/YEAR . . . . . . . . . . .

## THIS MONTH GOALS

## WEEKLY PRIORITIES

*W1*

*W2*

*W3*

*W4*

## OTHER TASKS

## MONTHLY AFFIRMATION

## REVIEW OF THE MONTH

## NOTES

# *WATER CHALLENGE*

MONTH/YEAR..................

| DAYS | WATER | DAYS | WATER |
|:---:|:---:|:---:|:---:|
| 01 | ▭▭▭▭▭▭▭▭ | 16 | ▭▭▭▭▭▭▭▭ |
| 02 | ▭▭▭▭▭▭▭▭ | 17 | ▭▭▭▭▭▭▭▭ |
| 03 | ▭▭▭▭▭▭▭▭ | 18 | ▭▭▭▭▭▭▭▭ |
| 04 | ▭▭▭▭▭▭▭▭ | 19 | ▭▭▭▭▭▭▭▭ |
| 05 | ▭▭▭▭▭▭▭▭ | 20 | ▭▭▭▭▭▭▭▭ |
| 06 | ▭▭▭▭▭▭▭▭ | 21 | ▭▭▭▭▭▭▭▭ |
| 07 | ▭▭▭▭▭▭▭▭ | 22 | ▭▭▭▭▭▭▭▭ |
| 08 | ▭▭▭▭▭▭▭▭ | 23 | ▭▭▭▭▭▭▭▭ |
| 09 | ▭▭▭▭▭▭▭▭ | 24 | ▭▭▭▭▭▭▭▭ |
| 10 | ▭▭▭▭▭▭▭▭ | 25 | ▭▭▭▭▭▭▭▭ |
| 11 | ▭▭▭▭▭▭▭▭ | 26 | ▭▭▭▭▭▭▭▭ |
| 12 | ▭▭▭▭▭▭▭▭ | 27 | ▭▭▭▭▭▭▭▭ |
| 13 | ▭▭▭▭▭▭▭▭ | 28 | ▭▭▭▭▭▭▭▭ |
| 14 | ▭▭▭▭▭▭▭▭ | 29 | ▭▭▭▭▭▭▭▭ |
| 15 | ▭▭▭▭▭▭▭▭ | 30 | ▭▭▭▭▭▭▭▭ |

# BODY PROGRESS TRACKER
## MONTH/YEAR

### WAIST

Week 1: ___________
Week 2: ___________
Week 3: ___________
Week 4: ___________

### ARMS

Week 1: ___________
Week 2: ___________
Week 3: ___________
Week 4: ___________

### THIGHS

Week 1: ___________
Week 2: ___________
Week 3: ___________
Week 4: ___________

### HIPS

Week 1: ___________
Week 2: ___________
Week 3: ___________
Week 4: ___________

| Goal Tracker | Week 1: | Week 2: | Week 3: | Week 4: |
|---|---|---|---|---|
| DATE | | | | |
| ARMS | | | | |
| WAIST | | | | |
| HIPS | | | | |
| THIGHS | | | | |
| WEIGHT | | | | |

# BODY MEASUREMENTS TRACKER
## MONTH/YEAR

| | BEFORE | AFTER |
|---|---|---|
| DATE | | |
| CHEST | | |
| LEFT ARM | | |
| RIGHT ARM | | |
| WAIST | | |
| HIPS | | |
| LEFT THIGH | | |
| RIGHT THIGH | | |
| LEFT CALF | | |
| RIGHT CALF | | |
| WEIGHT | | |
| NOTES | | |

# BODY GOALS

MONTH/YEAR . . . . . . . . . . .

## THIS MONTH GOALS

## WEEKLY PRIORITIES

W1

W2

W3

W4

## OTHER TASKS

## MONTHLY AFFIRMATION

## REVIEW OF THE MONTH

## NOTES

# WATER CHALLENGE

MONTH/YEAR.................

| DAYS | WATER | DAYS | WATER |
|------|-------|------|-------|
| 01 | ▽ ▽ ▽ ▽ ▽ ▽ ▽ ▽ | 16 | ▽ ▽ ▽ ▽ ▽ ▽ ▽ ▽ |
| 02 | ▽ ▽ ▽ ▽ ▽ ▽ ▽ ▽ | 17 | ▽ ▽ ▽ ▽ ▽ ▽ ▽ ▽ |
| 03 | ▽ ▽ ▽ ▽ ▽ ▽ ▽ ▽ | 18 | ▽ ▽ ▽ ▽ ▽ ▽ ▽ ▽ |
| 04 | ▽ ▽ ▽ ▽ ▽ ▽ ▽ ▽ | 19 | ▽ ▽ ▽ ▽ ▽ ▽ ▽ ▽ |
| 05 | ▽ ▽ ▽ ▽ ▽ ▽ ▽ ▽ | 20 | ▽ ▽ ▽ ▽ ▽ ▽ ▽ ▽ |
| 06 | ▽ ▽ ▽ ▽ ▽ ▽ ▽ ▽ | 21 | ▽ ▽ ▽ ▽ ▽ ▽ ▽ ▽ |
| 07 | ▽ ▽ ▽ ▽ ▽ ▽ ▽ ▽ | 22 | ▽ ▽ ▽ ▽ ▽ ▽ ▽ ▽ |
| 08 | ▽ ▽ ▽ ▽ ▽ ▽ ▽ ▽ | 23 | ▽ ▽ ▽ ▽ ▽ ▽ ▽ ▽ |
| 09 | ▽ ▽ ▽ ▽ ▽ ▽ ▽ ▽ | 24 | ▽ ▽ ▽ ▽ ▽ ▽ ▽ ▽ |
| 10 | ▽ ▽ ▽ ▽ ▽ ▽ ▽ ▽ | 25 | ▽ ▽ ▽ ▽ ▽ ▽ ▽ ▽ |
| 11 | ▽ ▽ ▽ ▽ ▽ ▽ ▽ ▽ | 26 | ▽ ▽ ▽ ▽ ▽ ▽ ▽ ▽ |
| 12 | ▽ ▽ ▽ ▽ ▽ ▽ ▽ ▽ | 27 | ▽ ▽ ▽ ▽ ▽ ▽ ▽ ▽ |
| 13 | ▽ ▽ ▽ ▽ ▽ ▽ ▽ ▽ | 28 | ▽ ▽ ▽ ▽ ▽ ▽ ▽ ▽ |
| 14 | ▽ ▽ ▽ ▽ ▽ ▽ ▽ ▽ | 29 | ▽ ▽ ▽ ▽ ▽ ▽ ▽ ▽ |
| 15 | ▽ ▽ ▽ ▽ ▽ ▽ ▽ ▽ | 30 | ▽ ▽ ▽ ▽ ▽ ▽ ▽ ▽ |

# BODY PROGRESS TRACKER

## MONTH/YEAR

### WAIST

Week 1: _____________

Week 2: _____________

Week 3: _____________

Week 4: _____________

### ARMS

Week 1: _____________

Week 2: _____________

Week 3: _____________

Week 4: _____________

### THIGHS

Week 1: _____________

Week 2: _____________

Week 3: _____________

Week 4: _____________

### HIPS

Week 1: _____________

Week 2: _____________

Week 3: _____________

Week 4: _____________

| Goal Tracker | Week 1: | Week 2: | Week 3: | Week 4: |
|---|---|---|---|---|
| DATE | | | | |
| ARMS | | | | |
| WAIST | | | | |
| HIPS | | | | |
| THIGHS | | | | |
| WEIGHT | | | | |

# BODY MEASUREMENTS TRACKER
## MONTH/YEAR

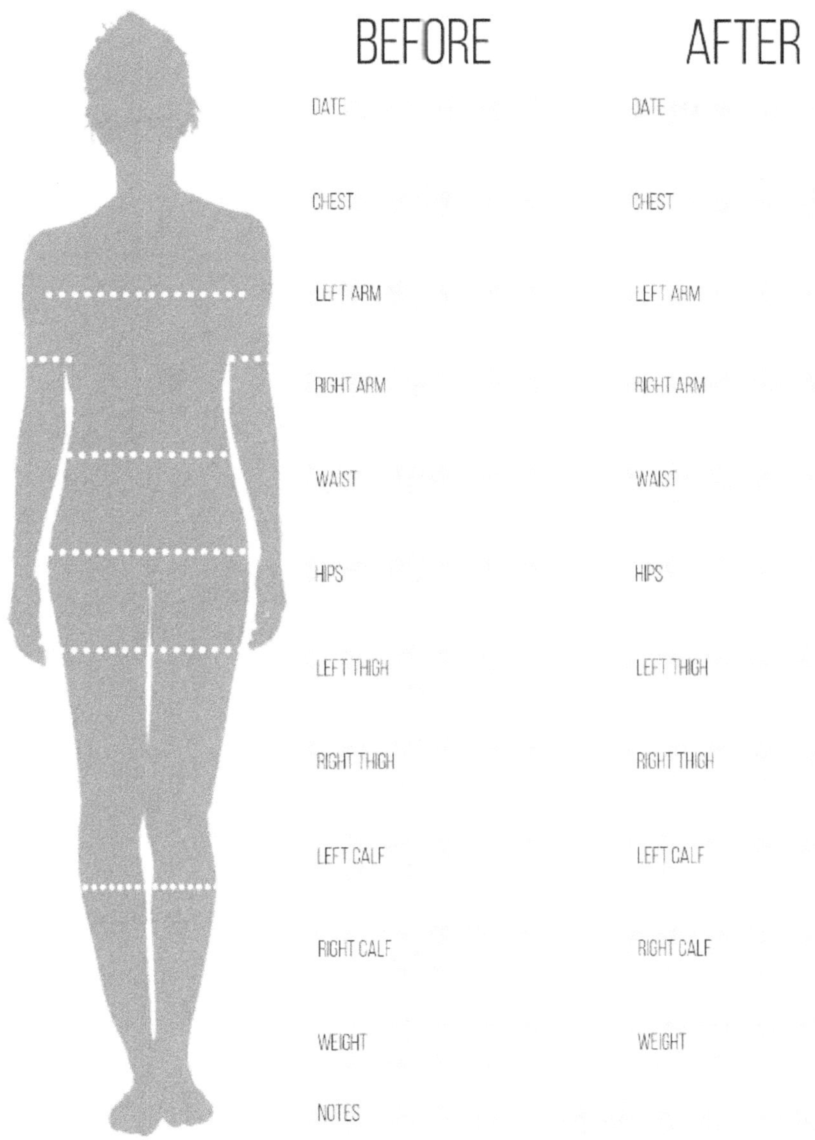

| BEFORE | AFTER |
| --- | --- |
| DATE | DATE |
| CHEST | CHEST |
| LEFT ARM | LEFT ARM |
| RIGHT ARM | RIGHT ARM |
| WAIST | WAIST |
| HIPS | HIPS |
| LEFT THIGH | LEFT THIGH |
| RIGHT THIGH | RIGHT THIGH |
| LEFT CALF | LEFT CALF |
| RIGHT CALF | RIGHT CALF |
| WEIGHT | WEIGHT |

NOTES

# BODY GOALS

MONTH/YEAR . . . . . . . . . . .

## THIS MONTH
## GOALS

## WEEKLY
## PRIORITIES

*W1*
*W2*
*W3*
*W4*

## OTHER TASKS

## MONTHLY
## AFFIRMATION

## REVIEW OF
## THE MONTH

## NOTES

# WATER CHALLENGE

MONTH/YEAR.................

| DAYS | WATER | DAYS | WATER |
|------|-------|------|-------|
| 01 | ▢▢▢▢▢▢▢▢ | 16 | ▢▢▢▢▢▢▢▢ |
| 02 | ▢▢▢▢▢▢▢▢ | 17 | ▢▢▢▢▢▢▢▢ |
| 03 | ▢▢▢▢▢▢▢▢ | 18 | ▢▢▢▢▢▢▢▢ |
| 04 | ▢▢▢▢▢▢▢▢ | 19 | ▢▢▢▢▢▢▢▢ |
| 05 | ▢▢▢▢▢▢▢▢ | 20 | ▢▢▢▢▢▢▢▢ |
| 06 | ▢▢▢▢▢▢▢▢ | 21 | ▢▢▢▢▢▢▢▢ |
| 07 | ▢▢▢▢▢▢▢▢ | 22 | ▢▢▢▢▢▢▢▢ |
| 08 | ▢▢▢▢▢▢▢▢ | 23 | ▢▢▢▢▢▢▢▢ |
| 09 | ▢▢▢▢▢▢▢▢ | 24 | ▢▢▢▢▢▢▢▢ |
| 10 | ▢▢▢▢▢▢▢▢ | 25 | ▢▢▢▢▢▢▢▢ |
| 11 | ▢▢▢▢▢▢▢▢ | 26 | ▢▢▢▢▢▢▢▢ |
| 12 | ▢▢▢▢▢▢▢▢ | 27 | ▢▢▢▢▢▢▢▢ |
| 13 | ▢▢▢▢▢▢▢▢ | 28 | ▢▢▢▢▢▢▢▢ |
| 14 | ▢▢▢▢▢▢▢▢ | 29 | ▢▢▢▢▢▢▢▢ |
| 15 | ▢▢▢▢▢▢▢▢ | 30 | ▢▢▢▢▢▢▢▢ |

# BODY PROGRESS TRACKER

## MONTH/YEAR

### WAIST

Week 1: _____________

Week 2: _____________

Week 3: _____________

Week 4: _____________

### ARMS

Week 1: _____________

Week 2: _____________

Week 3: _____________

Week 4: _____________

### THIGHS

Week 1: _____________

Week 2: _____________

Week 3: _____________

Week 4: _____________

### HIPS

Week 1: _____________

Week 2: _____________

Week 3: _____________

Week 4: _____________

| Goal Tracker | Week 1: | Week 2: | Week 3: | Week 4: |
|---|---|---|---|---|
| DATE | | | | |
| ARMS | | | | |
| WAIST | | | | |
| HIPS | | | | |
| THIGHS | | | | |
| WEIGHT | | | | |

# BODY MEASUREMENTS TRACKER
## MONTH/YEAR

| | BEFORE | AFTER |
|---|---|---|
| DATE | | |
| CHEST | | |
| LEFT ARM | | |
| RIGHT ARM | | |
| WAIST | | |
| HIPS | | |
| LEFT THIGH | | |
| RIGHT THIGH | | |
| LEFT CALF | | |
| RIGHT CALF | | |
| WEIGHT | | |
| NOTES | | |

# BODY GOALS

MONTH/YEAR . . . . . . . . . .

### THIS MONTH GOALS

### WEEKLY PRIORITIES

W1

W2

W3

W4

### OTHER TASKS

### MONTHLY AFFIRMATION

### REVIEW OF THE MONTH

### NOTES

# WATER CHALLENGE

MONTH/YEAR.................

| DAYS | WATER | DAYS | WATER |
|---|---|---|---|
| 01 | | 16 | |
| 02 | | 17 | |
| 03 | | 18 | |
| 04 | | 19 | |
| 05 | | 20 | |
| 06 | | 21 | |
| 07 | | 22 | |
| 08 | | 23 | |
| 09 | | 24 | |
| 10 | | 25 | |
| 11 | | 26 | |
| 12 | | 27 | |
| 13 | | 28 | |
| 14 | | 29 | |
| 15 | | 30 | |

# BODY PROGRESS TRACKER

## MONTH/YEAR

### WAIST

Week 1: _______________
Week 2: _______________
Week 3: _______________
Week 4: _______________

### ARMS

Week 1: _______________
Week 2: _______________
Week 3: _______________
Week 4: _______________

### THIGHS

Week 1: _______________
Week 2: _______________
Week 3: _______________
Week 4: _______________

### HIPS

Week 1: _______________
Week 2: _______________
Week 3: _______________
Week 4: _______________

| Goal Tracker | Week 1: | Week 2: | Week 3: | Week 4: |
|---|---|---|---|---|
| DATE | | | | |
| ARMS | | | | |
| WAIST | | | | |
| HIPS | | | | |
| THIGHS | | | | |
| WEIGHT | | | | |

# BODY MEASUREMENTS TRACKER
## MONTH/YEAR

|  | BEFORE | AFTER |
|---|---|---|
| DATE | | |
| CHEST | | |
| LEFT ARM | | |
| RIGHT ARM | | |
| WAIST | | |
| HIPS | | |
| LEFT THIGH | | |
| RIGHT THIGH | | |
| LEFT CALF | | |
| RIGHT CALF | | |
| WEIGHT | | |
| NOTES | | |

# BODY GOALS

MONTH/YEAR . . . . . . . . . . .

THIS MONTH
GOALS

WEEKLY
PRIORITIES

W1
W2
W3
W4

OTHER TASKS

MONTHLY
AFFIRMATION

REVIEW OF
THE MONTH

NOTES

# *WATER CHALLENGE*

MONTH/YEAR.................

| DAYS | WATER | DAYS | WATER |
|------|-------|------|-------|
| 01 | ▭▭▭▭▭▭▭▭ | 16 | ▭▭▭▭▭▭▭▭ |
| 02 | ▭▭▭▭▭▭▭▭ | 17 | ▭▭▭▭▭▭▭▭ |
| 03 | ▭▭▭▭▭▭▭▭ | 18 | ▭▭▭▭▭▭▭▭ |
| 04 | ▭▭▭▭▭▭▭▭ | 19 | ▭▭▭▭▭▭▭▭ |
| 05 | ▭▭▭▭▭▭▭▭ | 20 | ▭▭▭▭▭▭▭▭ |
| 06 | ▭▭▭▭▭▭▭▭ | 21 | ▭▭▭▭▭▭▭▭ |
| 07 | ▭▭▭▭▭▭▭▭ | 22 | ▭▭▭▭▭▭▭▭ |
| 08 | ▭▭▭▭▭▭▭▭ | 23 | ▭▭▭▭▭▭▭▭ |
| 09 | ▭▭▭▭▭▭▭▭ | 24 | ▭▭▭▭▭▭▭▭ |
| 10 | ▭▭▭▭▭▭▭▭ | 25 | ▭▭▭▭▭▭▭▭ |
| 11 | ▭▭▭▭▭▭▭▭ | 26 | ▭▭▭▭▭▭▭▭ |
| 12 | ▭▭▭▭▭▭▭▭ | 27 | ▭▭▭▭▭▭▭▭ |
| 13 | ▭▭▭▭▭▭▭▭ | 28 | ▭▭▭▭▭▭▭▭ |
| 14 | ▭▭▭▭▭▭▭▭ | 29 | ▭▭▭▭▭▭▭▭ |
| 15 | ▭▭▭▭▭▭▭▭ | 30 | ▭▭▭▭▭▭▭▭ |

# BODY PROGRESS TRACKER

MONTH/YEAR

## WAIST

Week 1: _______________

Week 2: _______________

Week 3: _______________

Week 4: _______________

## ARMS

Week 1: _______________

Week 2: _______________

Week 3: _______________

Week 4: _______________

## THIGHS

Week 1: _______________

Week 2: _______________

Week 3: _______________

Week 4: _______________

## HIPS

Week 1: _______________

Week 2: _______________

Week 3: _______________

Week 4: _______________

| Goal Tracker | Week 1: | Week 2: | Week 3: | Week 4: |
|---|---|---|---|---|
| DATE | | | | |
| ARMS | | | | |
| WAIST | | | | |
| HIPS | | | | |
| THIGHS | | | | |
| WEIGHT | | | | |

# BODY MEASUREMENTS TRACKER

## MONTH/YEAR

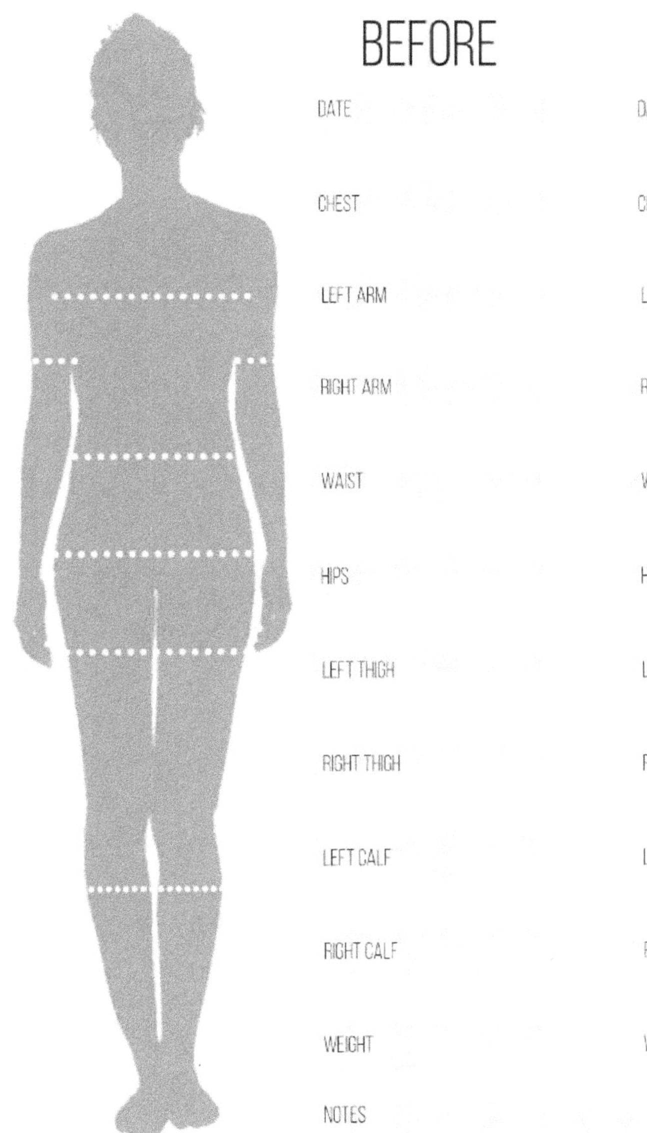

# BODY GOALS

MONTH/YEAR

## THIS MONTH
## GOALS

### WEEKLY PRIORITIES

*W1*

*W2*

*W3*

*W4*

### OTHER TASKS

### MONTHLY AFFIRMATION

### REVIEW OF THE MONTH

### NOTES

# *WATER CHALLENGE*

MONTH/YEAR.................

| DAYS | WATER | DAYS | WATER |
|---|---|---|---|
| 01 | ▽▽▽▽▽▽▽▽ | 16 | ▽▽▽▽▽▽▽▽ |
| 02 | ▽▽▽▽▽▽▽▽ | 17 | ▽▽▽▽▽▽▽▽ |
| 03 | ▽▽▽▽▽▽▽▽ | 18 | ▽▽▽▽▽▽▽▽ |
| 04 | ▽▽▽▽▽▽▽▽ | 19 | ▽▽▽▽▽▽▽▽ |
| 05 | ▽▽▽▽▽▽▽▽ | 20 | ▽▽▽▽▽▽▽▽ |
| 06 | ▽▽▽▽▽▽▽▽ | 21 | ▽▽▽▽▽▽▽▽ |
| 07 | ▽▽▽▽▽▽▽▽ | 22 | ▽▽▽▽▽▽▽▽ |
| 08 | ▽▽▽▽▽▽▽▽ | 23 | ▽▽▽▽▽▽▽▽ |
| 09 | ▽▽▽▽▽▽▽▽ | 24 | ▽▽▽▽▽▽▽▽ |
| 10 | ▽▽▽▽▽▽▽▽ | 25 | ▽▽▽▽▽▽▽▽ |
| 11 | ▽▽▽▽▽▽▽▽ | 26 | ▽▽▽▽▽▽▽▽ |
| 12 | ▽▽▽▽▽▽▽▽ | 27 | ▽▽▽▽▽▽▽▽ |
| 13 | ▽▽▽▽▽▽▽▽ | 28 | ▽▽▽▽▽▽▽▽ |
| 14 | ▽▽▽▽▽▽▽▽ | 29 | ▽▽▽▽▽▽▽▽ |
| 15 | ▽▽▽▽▽▽▽▽ | 30 | ▽▽▽▽▽▽▽▽ |

# BODY PROGRESS TRACKER

## MONTH/YEAR

### WAIST

Week 1: _______________

Week 2: _______________

Week 3: _______________

Week 4: _______________

### ARMS

Week 1: _______________

Week 2: _______________

Week 3: _______________

Week 4: _______________

### THIGHS

Week 1: _______________

Week 2: _______________

Week 3: _______________

Week 4: _______________

### HIPS

Week 1: _______________

Week 2: _______________

Week 3: _______________

Week 4: _______________

| Goal Tracker | Week 1: | Week 2: | Week 3: | Week 4: |
|---|---|---|---|---|
| DATE | | | | |
| ARMS | | | | |
| WAIST | | | | |
| HIPS | | | | |
| THIGHS | | | | |
| WEIGHT | | | | |

# BODY MEASUREMENTS TRACKER

## MONTH/YEAR

| BEFORE | AFTER |
|---|---|
| DATE | DATE |
| CHEST | CHEST |
| LEFT ARM | LEFT ARM |
| RIGHT ARM | RIGHT ARM |
| WAIST | WAIST |
| HIPS | HIPS |
| LEFT THIGH | LEFT THIGH |
| RIGHT THIGH | RIGHT THIGH |
| LEFT CALF | LEFT CALF |
| RIGHT CALF | RIGHT CALF |
| WEIGHT | WEIGHT |

NOTES

# BODY GOALS

MONTH/YEAR . . . . . . . . . .

## THIS MONTH GOALS

## WEEKLY PRIORITIES

*W1*
*W2*
*W3*
*W4*

## OTHER TASKS

## MONTHLY AFFIRMATION

## REVIEW OF THE MONTH

## NOTES

# WATER CHALLENGE

MONTH/YEAR.................

| DAYS | WATER | DAYS | WATER |
|------|-------|------|-------|
| 01 | ▽▽▽▽▽▽▽▽ | 16 | ▽▽▽▽▽▽▽▽ |
| 02 | ▽▽▽▽▽▽▽▽ | 17 | ▽▽▽▽▽▽▽▽ |
| 03 | ▽▽▽▽▽▽▽▽ | 18 | ▽▽▽▽▽▽▽▽ |
| 04 | ▽▽▽▽▽▽▽▽ | 19 | ▽▽▽▽▽▽▽▽ |
| 05 | ▽▽▽▽▽▽▽▽ | 20 | ▽▽▽▽▽▽▽▽ |
| 06 | ▽▽▽▽▽▽▽▽ | 21 | ▽▽▽▽▽▽▽▽ |
| 07 | ▽▽▽▽▽▽▽▽ | 22 | ▽▽▽▽▽▽▽▽ |
| 08 | ▽▽▽▽▽▽▽▽ | 23 | ▽▽▽▽▽▽▽▽ |
| 09 | ▽▽▽▽▽▽▽▽ | 24 | ▽▽▽▽▽▽▽▽ |
| 10 | ▽▽▽▽▽▽▽▽ | 25 | ▽▽▽▽▽▽▽▽ |
| 11 | ▽▽▽▽▽▽▽▽ | 26 | ▽▽▽▽▽▽▽▽ |
| 12 | ▽▽▽▽▽▽▽▽ | 27 | ▽▽▽▽▽▽▽▽ |
| 13 | ▽▽▽▽▽▽▽▽ | 28 | ▽▽▽▽▽▽▽▽ |
| 14 | ▽▽▽▽▽▽▽▽ | 29 | ▽▽▽▽▽▽▽▽ |
| 15 | ▽▽▽▽▽▽▽▽ | 30 | ▽▽▽▽▽▽▽▽ |

# BODY PROGRESS TRACKER

## MONTH/YEAR

### WAIST

Week 1: _______________

Week 2: _______________

Week 3: _______________

Week 4: _______________

### ARMS

Week 1: _______________

Week 2: _______________

Week 3: _______________

Week 4: _______________

### THIGHS

Week 1: _______________

Week 2: _______________

Week 3: _______________

Week 4: _______________

### HIPS

Week 1: _______________

Week 2: _______________

Week 3: _______________

Week 4: _______________

| Goal Tracker | Week 1: | Week 2: | Week 3: | Week 4: |
|---|---|---|---|---|
| DATE | | | | |
| ARMS | | | | |
| WAIST | | | | |
| HIPS | | | | |
| THIGHS | | | | |
| WEIGHT | | | | |

# BODY MEASUREMENTS TRACKER

## MONTH/YEAR

| | BEFORE | AFTER |
| --- | --- | --- |
| DATE | | |
| CHEST | | |
| LEFT ARM | | |
| RIGHT ARM | | |
| WAIST | | |
| HIPS | | |
| LEFT THIGH | | |
| RIGHT THIGH | | |
| LEFT CALF | | |
| RIGHT CALF | | |
| WEIGHT | | |
| NOTES | | |

# BODY GOALS

MONTH/YEAR . . . . . . . . . .

### THIS MONTH GOALS

### WEEKLY PRIORITIES

*W1*
*W2*
*W3*
*W4*

### OTHER TASKS

### MONTHLY AFFIRMATION

### REVIEW OF THE MONTH

### NOTES

# WATER CHALLENGE

MONTH/YEAR.................

| DAYS | WATER | DAYS | WATER |
|------|-------|------|-------|
| 01 | ▾ ▾ ▾ ▾ ▾ ▾ ▾ ▾ | 16 | ▾ ▾ ▾ ▾ ▾ ▾ ▾ ▾ |
| 02 | ▾ ▾ ▾ ▾ ▾ ▾ ▾ ▾ | 17 | ▾ ▾ ▾ ▾ ▾ ▾ ▾ ▾ |
| 03 | ▾ ▾ ▾ ▾ ▾ ▾ ▾ ▾ | 18 | ▾ ▾ ▾ ▾ ▾ ▾ ▾ ▾ |
| 04 | ▾ ▾ ▾ ▾ ▾ ▾ ▾ ▾ | 19 | ▾ ▾ ▾ ▾ ▾ ▾ ▾ ▾ |
| 05 | ▾ ▾ ▾ ▾ ▾ ▾ ▾ ▾ | 20 | ▾ ▾ ▾ ▾ ▾ ▾ ▾ ▾ |
| 06 | ▾ ▾ ▾ ▾ ▾ ▾ ▾ ▾ | 21 | ▾ ▾ ▾ ▾ ▾ ▾ ▾ ▾ |
| 07 | ▾ ▾ ▾ ▾ ▾ ▾ ▾ ▾ | 22 | ▾ ▾ ▾ ▾ ▾ ▾ ▾ ▾ |
| 08 | ▾ ▾ ▾ ▾ ▾ ▾ ▾ ▾ | 23 | ▾ ▾ ▾ ▾ ▾ ▾ ▾ ▾ |
| 09 | ▾ ▾ ▾ ▾ ▾ ▾ ▾ ▾ | 24 | ▾ ▾ ▾ ▾ ▾ ▾ ▾ ▾ |
| 10 | ▾ ▾ ▾ ▾ ▾ ▾ ▾ ▾ | 25 | ▾ ▾ ▾ ▾ ▾ ▾ ▾ ▾ |
| 11 | ▾ ▾ ▾ ▾ ▾ ▾ ▾ ▾ | 26 | ▾ ▾ ▾ ▾ ▾ ▾ ▾ ▾ |
| 12 | ▾ ▾ ▾ ▾ ▾ ▾ ▾ ▾ | 27 | ▾ ▾ ▾ ▾ ▾ ▾ ▾ ▾ |
| 13 | ▾ ▾ ▾ ▾ ▾ ▾ ▾ ▾ | 28 | ▾ ▾ ▾ ▾ ▾ ▾ ▾ ▾ |
| 14 | ▾ ▾ ▾ ▾ ▾ ▾ ▾ ▾ | 29 | ▾ ▾ ▾ ▾ ▾ ▾ ▾ ▾ |
| 15 | ▾ ▾ ▾ ▾ ▾ ▾ ▾ ▾ | 30 | ▾ ▾ ▾ ▾ ▾ ▾ ▾ ▾ |

# BODY PROGRESS TRACKER

## MONTH/YEAR

### WAIST

Week 1: _______________

Week 2: _______________

Week 3: _______________

Week 4: _______________

### ARMS

Week 1: _______________

Week 2: _______________

Week 3: _______________

Week 4: _______________

### THIGHS

Week 1: _______________

Week 2: _______________

Week 3: _______________

Week 4: _______________

### HIPS

Week 1: _______________

Week 2: _______________

Week 3: _______________

Week 4: _______________

| Goal Tracker | Week 1: | Week 2: | Week 3: | Week 4: |
|---|---|---|---|---|
| DATE | | | | |
| ARMS | | | | |
| WAIST | | | | |
| HIPS | | | | |
| THIGHS | | | | |
| WEIGHT | | | | |

# BODY MEASUREMENTS TRACKER
## MONTH/YEAR

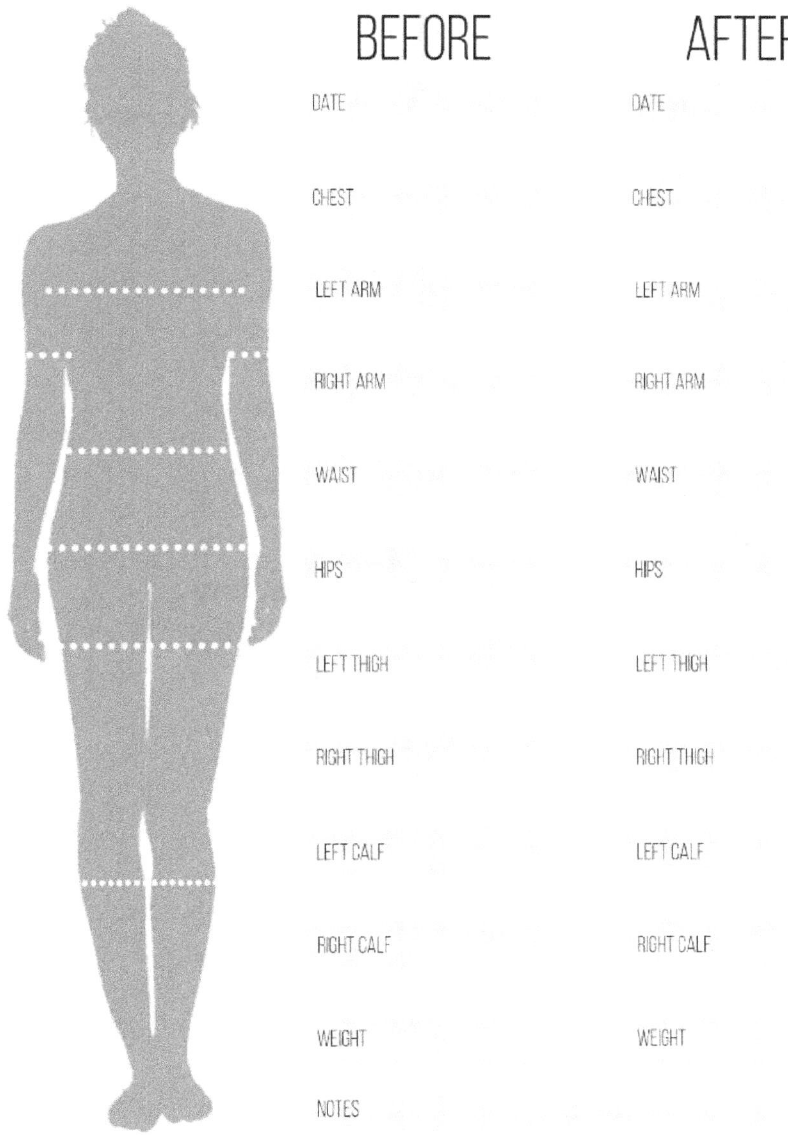

# BODY GOALS

MONTH/YEAR . . . . . . . . . . .

## THIS MONTH
## GOALS

## WEEKLY
## PRIORITIES

W1
W2
W3
W4

## OTHER TASKS

## MONTHLY
## AFFIRMATION

## REVIEW OF
## THE MONTH

## NOTES

# WATER CHALLENGE

MONTH/YEAR.................

| DAYS | WATER | DAYS | WATER |
|------|-------|------|-------|
| 01 | | 16 | |
| 02 | | 17 | |
| 03 | | 18 | |
| 04 | | 19 | |
| 05 | | 20 | |
| 06 | | 21 | |
| 07 | | 22 | |
| 08 | | 23 | |
| 09 | | 24 | |
| 10 | | 25 | |
| 11 | | 26 | |
| 12 | | 27 | |
| 13 | | 28 | |
| 14 | | 29 | |
| 15 | | 30 | |

# BODY PROGRESS TRACKER

## MONTH/YEAR

### WAIST

Week 1: _____________

Week 2: _____________

Week 3: _____________

Week 4: _____________

### ARMS

Week 1: _____________

Week 2: _____________

Week 3: _____________

Week 4: _____________

### THIGHS

Week 1: _____________

Week 2: _____________

Week 3: _____________

Week 4: _____________

### HIPS

Week 1: _____________

Week 2: _____________

Week 3: _____________

Week 4: _____________

| Goal Tracker | Week 1: | Week 2: | Week 3: | Week 4: |
|---|---|---|---|---|
| DATE | | | | |
| ARMS | | | | |
| WAIST | | | | |
| HIPS | | | | |
| THIGHS | | | | |
| WEIGHT | | | | |

# BODY MEASUREMENTS TRACKER

## MONTH/YEAR

| | BEFORE | AFTER |
|---|---|---|
| DATE | | |
| CHEST | | |
| LEFT ARM | | |
| RIGHT ARM | | |
| WAIST | | |
| HIPS | | |
| LEFT THIGH | | |
| RIGHT THIGH | | |
| LEFT CALF | | |
| RIGHT CALF | | |
| WEIGHT | | |
| NOTES | | |

# BODY GOALS

MONTH/YEAR . . . . . . . . . . .

THIS MONTH
GOALS

WEEKLY
PRIORITIES

*W1*
*W2*
*W3*
*W4*

OTHER TASKS

MONTHLY
AFFIRMATION

REVIEW OF
THE MONTH

NOTES

# WATER CHALLENGE

MONTH/YEAR.................

| DAYS | WATER | DAYS | WATER |
|:---:|:---:|:---:|:---:|
| 01 | | 16 | |
| 02 | | 17 | |
| 03 | | 18 | |
| 04 | | 19 | |
| 05 | | 20 | |
| 06 | | 21 | |
| 07 | | 22 | |
| 08 | | 23 | |
| 09 | | 24 | |
| 10 | | 25 | |
| 11 | | 26 | |
| 12 | | 27 | |
| 13 | | 28 | |
| 14 | | 29 | |
| 15 | | 30 | |

# BODY PROGRESS TRACKER

## MONTH/YEAR

### WAIST

Week 1: _____________

Week 2: _____________

Week 3: _____________

Week 4: _____________

### ARMS

Week 1: _____________

Week 2: _____________

Week 3: _____________

Week 4: _____________

### THIGHS

Week 1: _____________

Week 2: _____________

Week 3: _____________

Week 4: _____________

### HIPS

Week 1: _____________

Week 2: _____________

Week 3: _____________

Week 4: _____________

| Goal Tracker | Week 1: | Week 2: | Week 3: | Week 4: |
|---|---|---|---|---|
| DATE | | | | |
| ARMS | | | | |
| WAIST | | | | |
| HIPS | | | | |
| THIGHS | | | | |
| WEIGHT | | | | |

# BODY MEASUREMENTS TRACKER
## MONTH/YEAR

| | BEFORE | AFTER |
|---|---|---|
| DATE | | |
| CHEST | | |
| LEFT ARM | | |
| RIGHT ARM | | |
| WAIST | | |
| HIPS | | |
| LEFT THIGH | | |
| RIGHT THIGH | | |
| LEFT CALF | | |
| RIGHT CALF | | |
| WEIGHT | | |
| NOTES | | |

# BODY GOALS

MONTH/YEAR . . . . . . . . . .

### THIS MONTH
### GOALS

### WEEKLY
### PRIORITIES

*W1*

*W2*

*W3*

*W4*

### OTHER TASKS

### MONTHLY
### AFFIRMATION

### REVIEW OF
### THE MONTH

### NOTES

# WATER CHALLENGE

MONTH/YEAR..................

| DAYS | WATER | DAYS | WATER |
|------|-------|------|-------|
| 01 | | 16 | |
| 02 | | 17 | |
| 03 | | 18 | |
| 04 | | 19 | |
| 05 | | 20 | |
| 06 | | 21 | |
| 07 | | 22 | |
| 08 | | 23 | |
| 09 | | 24 | |
| 10 | | 25 | |
| 11 | | 26 | |
| 12 | | 27 | |
| 13 | | 28 | |
| 14 | | 29 | |
| 15 | | 30 | |

# BODY PROGRESS TRACKER

## MONTH/YEAR

### WAIST

Week 1: _______________

Week 2: _______________

Week 3: _______________

Week 4: _______________

### ARMS

Week 1: _______________

Week 2: _______________

Week 3: _______________

Week 4: _______________

### THIGHS

Week 1: _______________

Week 2: _______________

Week 3: _______________

Week 4: _______________

### HIPS

Week 1: _______________

Week 2: _______________

Week 3: _______________

Week 4: _______________

| Goal Tracker | Week 1: | Week 2: | Week 3: | Week 4: |
|---|---|---|---|---|
| DATE | | | | |
| ARMS | | | | |
| WAIST | | | | |
| HIPS | | | | |
| THIGHS | | | | |
| WEIGHT | | | | |

# BODY MEASUREMENTS TRACKER

## MONTH/YEAR

|  | BEFORE | AFTER |
|---|---|---|
| DATE | | |
| CHEST | | |
| LEFT ARM | | |
| RIGHT ARM | | |
| WAIST | | |
| HIPS | | |
| LEFT THIGH | | |
| RIGHT THIGH | | |
| LEFT CALF | | |
| RIGHT CALF | | |
| WEIGHT | | |
| NOTES | | |

# BODY GOALS

MONTH/YEAR . . . . . . . . . . .

## THIS MONTH
## GOALS

## WEEKLY
## PRIORITIES

**W1**

**W2**

**W3**

**W4**

## OTHER TASKS

## MONTHLY
## AFFIRMATION

## REVIEW OF
## THE MONTH

## NOTES

# WATER CHALLENGE

MONTH/YEAR.................

| DAYS | WATER | DAYS | WATER |
|------|-------|------|-------|
| 01 | ▭▭▭▭▭▭▭▭ | 16 | ▭▭▭▭▭▭▭▭ |
| 02 | ▭▭▭▭▭▭▭▭ | 17 | ▭▭▭▭▭▭▭▭ |
| 03 | ▭▭▭▭▭▭▭▭ | 18 | ▭▭▭▭▭▭▭▭ |
| 04 | ▭▭▭▭▭▭▭▭ | 19 | ▭▭▭▭▭▭▭▭ |
| 05 | ▭▭▭▭▭▭▭▭ | 20 | ▭▭▭▭▭▭▭▭ |
| 06 | ▭▭▭▭▭▭▭▭ | 21 | ▭▭▭▭▭▭▭▭ |
| 07 | ▭▭▭▭▭▭▭▭ | 22 | ▭▭▭▭▭▭▭▭ |
| 08 | ▭▭▭▭▭▭▭▭ | 23 | ▭▭▭▭▭▭▭▭ |
| 09 | ▭▭▭▭▭▭▭▭ | 24 | ▭▭▭▭▭▭▭▭ |
| 10 | ▭▭▭▭▭▭▭▭ | 25 | ▭▭▭▭▭▭▭▭ |
| 11 | ▭▭▭▭▭▭▭▭ | 26 | ▭▭▭▭▭▭▭▭ |
| 12 | ▭▭▭▭▭▭▭▭ | 27 | ▭▭▭▭▭▭▭▭ |
| 13 | ▭▭▭▭▭▭▭▭ | 28 | ▭▭▭▭▭▭▭▭ |
| 14 | ▭▭▭▭▭▭▭▭ | 29 | ▭▭▭▭▭▭▭▭ |
| 15 | ▭▭▭▭▭▭▭▭ | 30 | ▭▭▭▭▭▭▭▭ |

# BODY PROGRESS TRACKER

## MONTH/YEAR

### WAIST

Week 1: ___________

Week 2: ___________

Week 3: ___________

Week 4: ___________

### THIGHS

Week 1: ___________

Week 2: ___________

Week 3: ___________

Week 4: ___________

### ARMS

Week 1: ___________

Week 2: ___________

Week 3: ___________

Week 4: ___________

### HIPS

Week 1: ___________

Week 2: ___________

Week 3: ___________

Week 4: ___________

| Goal Tracker | Week 1: | Week 2: | Week 3: | Week 4: |
| --- | --- | --- | --- | --- |
| DATE | | | | |
| ARMS | | | | |
| WAIST | | | | |
| HIPS | | | | |
| THIGHS | | | | |
| WEIGHT | | | | |

# BODY MEASUREMENTS TRACKER
## MONTH/YEAR

BEFORE

AFTER

DATE

CHEST

LEFT ARM

RIGHT ARM

WAIST

HIPS

LEFT THIGH

RIGHT THIGH

LEFT CALF

RIGHT CALF

WEIGHT

NOTES

# BODY GOALS

MONTH/YEAR . . . . . . . . . . .

THIS MONTH
GOALS

WEEKLY
PRIORITIES

W1
W2
W3
W4

OTHER TASKS

MONTHLY
AFFIRMATION

REVIEW OF
THE MONTH

NOTES

# WATER CHALLENGE

MONTH/YEAR.................

| DAYS | WATER | DAYS | WATER |
|:---:|:---:|:---:|:---:|
| 01 | ▽▽▽▽▽▽▽▽ | 16 | ▽▽▽▽▽▽▽▽ |
| 02 | ▽▽▽▽▽▽▽▽ | 17 | ▽▽▽▽▽▽▽▽ |
| 03 | ▽▽▽▽▽▽▽▽ | 18 | ▽▽▽▽▽▽▽▽ |
| 04 | ▽▽▽▽▽▽▽▽ | 19 | ▽▽▽▽▽▽▽▽ |
| 05 | ▽▽▽▽▽▽▽▽ | 20 | ▽▽▽▽▽▽▽▽ |
| 06 | ▽▽▽▽▽▽▽▽ | 21 | ▽▽▽▽▽▽▽▽ |
| 07 | ▽▽▽▽▽▽▽▽ | 22 | ▽▽▽▽▽▽▽▽ |
| 08 | ▽▽▽▽▽▽▽▽ | 23 | ▽▽▽▽▽▽▽▽ |
| 09 | ▽▽▽▽▽▽▽▽ | 24 | ▽▽▽▽▽▽▽▽ |
| 10 | ▽▽▽▽▽▽▽▽ | 25 | ▽▽▽▽▽▽▽▽ |
| 11 | ▽▽▽▽▽▽▽▽ | 26 | ▽▽▽▽▽▽▽▽ |
| 12 | ▽▽▽▽▽▽▽▽ | 27 | ▽▽▽▽▽▽▽▽ |
| 13 | ▽▽▽▽▽▽▽▽ | 28 | ▽▽▽▽▽▽▽▽ |
| 14 | ▽▽▽▽▽▽▽▽ | 29 | ▽▽▽▽▽▽▽▽ |
| 15 | ▽▽▽▽▽▽▽▽ | 30 | ▽▽▽▽▽▽▽▽ |

# BODY PROGRESS TRACKER

## MONTH/YEAR

### WAIST

Week 1: _______________

Week 2: _______________

Week 3: _______________

Week 4: _______________

### ARMS

Week 1: _______________

Week 2: _______________

Week 3: _______________

Week 4: _______________

### THIGHS

Week 1: _______________

Week 2: _______________

Week 3: _______________

Week 4: _______________

### HIPS

Week 1: _______________

Week 2: _______________

Week 3: _______________

Week 4: _______________

| Goal Tracker | Week 1: | Week 2: | Week 3: | Week 4: |
|---|---|---|---|---|
| DATE | | | | |
| ARMS | | | | |
| WAIST | | | | |
| HIPS | | | | |
| THIGHS | | | | |
| WEIGHT | | | | |

# BODY MEASUREMENTS TRACKER
## MONTH/YEAR

| | BEFORE | AFTER |
|---|---|---|
| DATE | | |
| CHEST | | |
| LEFT ARM | | |
| RIGHT ARM | | |
| WAIST | | |
| HIPS | | |
| LEFT THIGH | | |
| RIGHT THIGH | | |
| LEFT CALF | | |
| RIGHT CALF | | |
| WEIGHT | | |
| NOTES | | |

# BODY GOALS

MONTH/YEAR ............

## THIS MONTH GOALS

## WEEKLY PRIORITIES

*W1*

*W2*

*W3*

*W4*

## OTHER TASKS

## MONTHLY AFFIRMATION

## REVIEW OF THE MONTH

## NOTES

# *WATER CHALLENGE*

MONTH/YEAR.................

| DAYS | WATER | DAYS | WATER |
|---|---|---|---|
| 01 | ▽▽▽▽▽▽▽▽ | 16 | ▽▽▽▽▽▽▽▽ |
| 02 | ▽▽▽▽▽▽▽▽ | 17 | ▽▽▽▽▽▽▽▽ |
| 03 | ▽▽▽▽▽▽▽▽ | 18 | ▽▽▽▽▽▽▽▽ |
| 04 | ▽▽▽▽▽▽▽▽ | 19 | ▽▽▽▽▽▽▽▽ |
| 05 | ▽▽▽▽▽▽▽▽ | 20 | ▽▽▽▽▽▽▽▽ |
| 06 | ▽▽▽▽▽▽▽▽ | 21 | ▽▽▽▽▽▽▽▽ |
| 07 | ▽▽▽▽▽▽▽▽ | 22 | ▽▽▽▽▽▽▽▽ |
| 08 | ▽▽▽▽▽▽▽▽ | 23 | ▽▽▽▽▽▽▽▽ |
| 09 | ▽▽▽▽▽▽▽▽ | 24 | ▽▽▽▽▽▽▽▽ |
| 10 | ▽▽▽▽▽▽▽▽ | 25 | ▽▽▽▽▽▽▽▽ |
| 11 | ▽▽▽▽▽▽▽▽ | 26 | ▽▽▽▽▽▽▽▽ |
| 12 | ▽▽▽▽▽▽▽▽ | 27 | ▽▽▽▽▽▽▽▽ |
| 13 | ▽▽▽▽▽▽▽▽ | 28 | ▽▽▽▽▽▽▽▽ |
| 14 | ▽▽▽▽▽▽▽▽ | 29 | ▽▽▽▽▽▽▽▽ |
| 15 | ▽▽▽▽▽▽▽▽ | 30 | ▽▽▽▽▽▽▽▽ |

# BODY PROGRESS TRACKER

## MONTH/YEAR

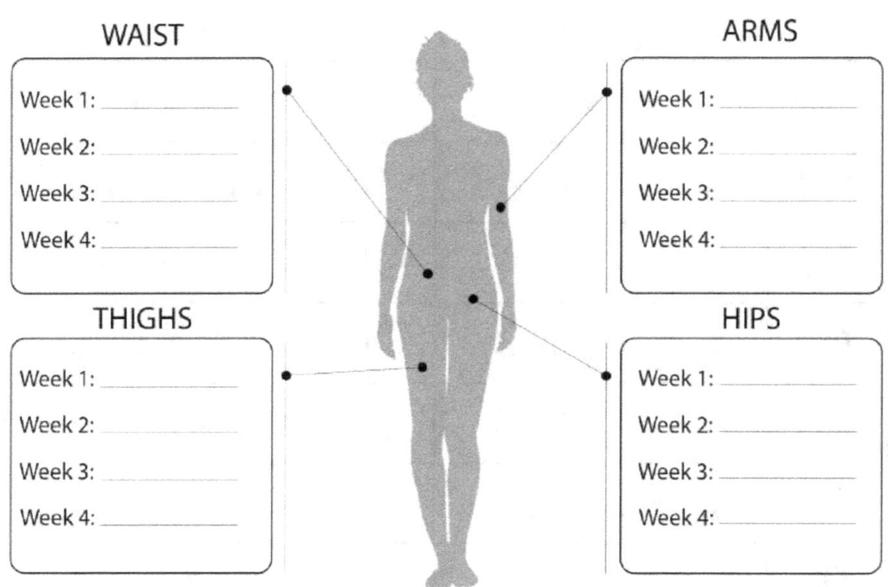



| Goal Tracker | Week 1: | Week 2: | Week 3: | Week 4: |
|---|---|---|---|---|
| DATE | | | | |
| ARMS | | | | |
| WAIST | | | | |
| HIPS | | | | |
| THIGHS | | | | |
| WEIGHT | | | | |

# BODY MEASUREMENTS TRACKER
## MONTH/YEAR

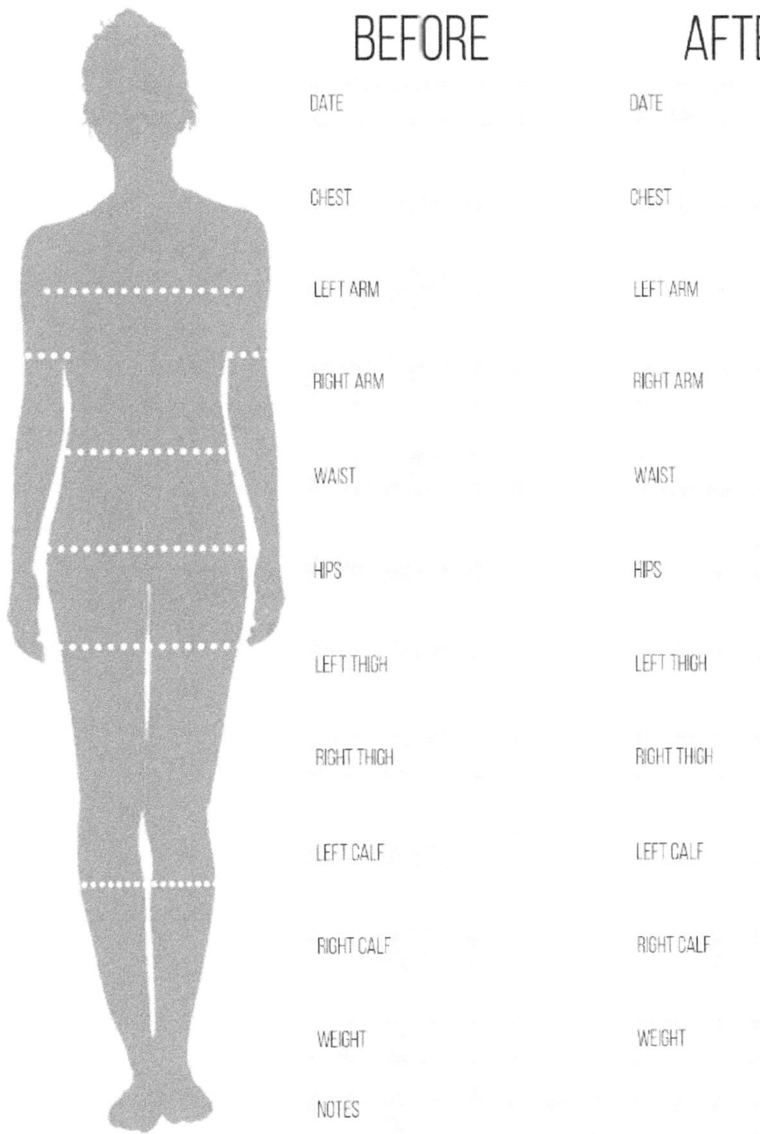

# BODY GOALS

MONTH/YEAR . . . . . . . . . . .

### THIS MONTH GOALS

### WEEKLY PRIORITIES

**W1**

**W2**

**W3**

**W4**

### OTHER TASKS

### MONTHLY AFFIRMATION

### REVIEW OF THE MONTH

### NOTES

# WATER CHALLENGE

MONTH/YEAR................

| DAYS | WATER | DAYS | WATER |
|---|---|---|---|
| 01 | ▽▽▽▽▽▽▽▽ | 16 | ▽▽▽▽▽▽▽▽ |
| 02 | ▽▽▽▽▽▽▽▽ | 17 | ▽▽▽▽▽▽▽▽ |
| 03 | ▽▽▽▽▽▽▽▽ | 18 | ▽▽▽▽▽▽▽▽ |
| 04 | ▽▽▽▽▽▽▽▽ | 19 | ▽▽▽▽▽▽▽▽ |
| 05 | ▽▽▽▽▽▽▽▽ | 20 | ▽▽▽▽▽▽▽▽ |
| 06 | ▽▽▽▽▽▽▽▽ | 21 | ▽▽▽▽▽▽▽▽ |
| 07 | ▽▽▽▽▽▽▽▽ | 22 | ▽▽▽▽▽▽▽▽ |
| 08 | ▽▽▽▽▽▽▽▽ | 23 | ▽▽▽▽▽▽▽▽ |
| 09 | ▽▽▽▽▽▽▽▽ | 24 | ▽▽▽▽▽▽▽▽ |
| 10 | ▽▽▽▽▽▽▽▽ | 25 | ▽▽▽▽▽▽▽▽ |
| 11 | ▽▽▽▽▽▽▽▽ | 26 | ▽▽▽▽▽▽▽▽ |
| 12 | ▽▽▽▽▽▽▽▽ | 27 | ▽▽▽▽▽▽▽▽ |
| 13 | ▽▽▽▽▽▽▽▽ | 28 | ▽▽▽▽▽▽▽▽ |
| 14 | ▽▽▽▽▽▽▽▽ | 29 | ▽▽▽▽▽▽▽▽ |
| 15 | ▽▽▽▽▽▽▽▽ | 30 | ▽▽▽▽▽▽▽▽ |

# BODY PROGRESS TRACKER

## MONTH/YEAR ..............

### WAIST

Week 1: _______________

Week 2: _______________

Week 3: _______________

Week 4: _______________

### ARMS

Week 1: _______________

Week 2: _______________

Week 3: _______________

Week 4: _______________

### THIGHS

Week 1: _______________

Week 2: _______________

Week 3: _______________

Week 4: _______________

### HIPS

Week 1: _______________

Week 2: _______________

Week 3: _______________

Week 4: _______________

| Goal Tracker | Week 1: | Week 2: | Week 3: | Week 4: |
|---|---|---|---|---|
| DATE | | | | |
| ARMS | | | | |
| WAIST | | | | |
| HIPS | | | | |
| THIGHS | | | | |
| WEIGHT | | | | |

# BODY MEASUREMENTS TRACKER
## MONTH/YEAR

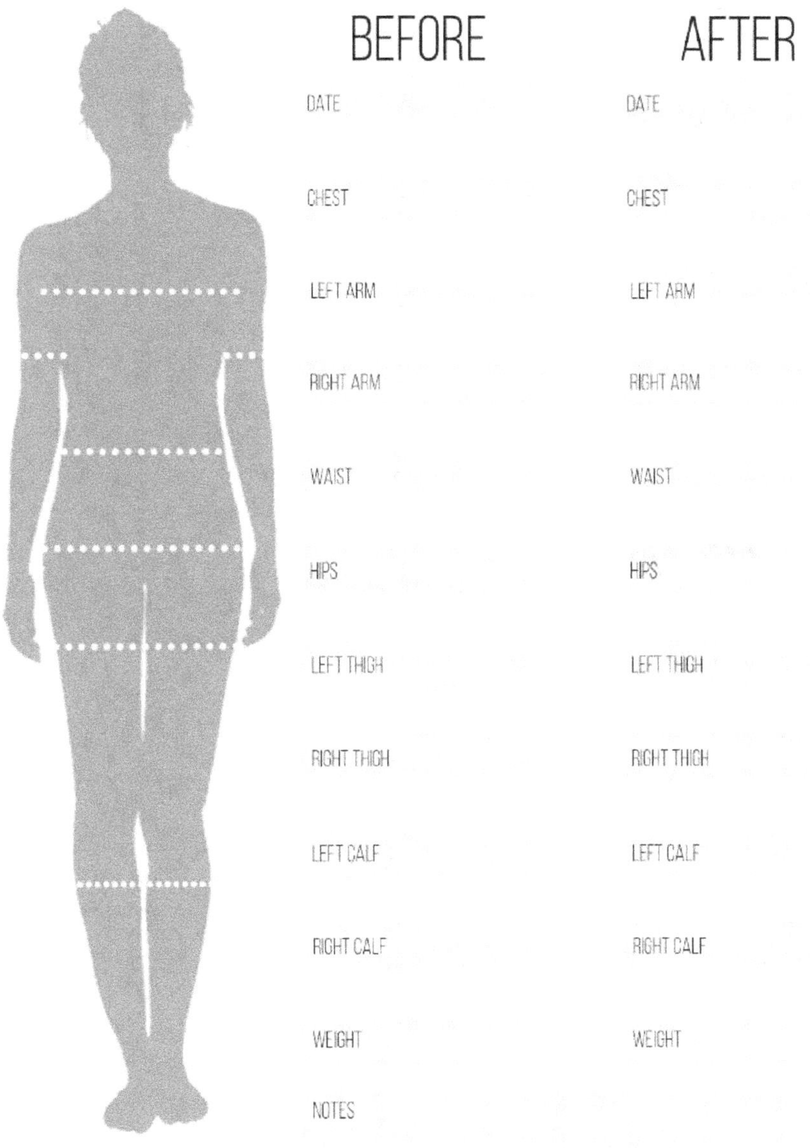

# BODY GOALS

MONTH/YEAR . . . . . . . . . . .

## THIS MONTH GOALS

## WEEKLY PRIORITIES

W1

W2

W3

W4

## OTHER TASKS

## MONTHLY AFFIRMATION

## REVIEW OF THE MONTH

## NOTES

# WATER CHALLENGE

MONTH/YEAR.................

| DAYS | WATER | DAYS | WATER |
|------|-------|------|-------|
| 01 |  | 16 |  |
| 02 |  | 17 |  |
| 03 |  | 18 |  |
| 04 |  | 19 |  |
| 05 |  | 20 |  |
| 06 |  | 21 |  |
| 07 |  | 22 |  |
| 08 |  | 23 |  |
| 09 |  | 24 |  |
| 10 |  | 25 |  |
| 11 |  | 26 |  |
| 12 |  | 27 |  |
| 13 |  | 28 |  |
| 14 |  | 29 |  |
| 15 |  | 30 |  |

# BODY PROGRESS TRACKER

## MONTH/YEAR

### WAIST

Week 1: _____________

Week 2: _____________

Week 3: _____________

Week 4: _____________

### THIGHS

Week 1: _____________

Week 2: _____________

Week 3: _____________

Week 4: _____________

### ARMS

Week 1: _____________

Week 2: _____________

Week 3: _____________

Week 4: _____________

### HIPS

Week 1: _____________

Week 2: _____________

Week 3: _____________

Week 4: _____________

| Goal Tracker | Week 1: | Week 2: | Week 3: | Week 4: |
|---|---|---|---|---|
| DATE | | | | |
| ARMS | | | | |
| WAIST | | | | |
| HIPS | | | | |
| THIGHS | | | | |
| WEIGHT | | | | |

# BODY MEASUREMENTS TRACKER

## MONTH/YEAR

| | BEFORE | AFTER |
|---|---|---|
| DATE | | |
| CHEST | | |
| LEFT ARM | | |
| RIGHT ARM | | |
| WAIST | | |
| HIPS | | |
| LEFT THIGH | | |
| RIGHT THIGH | | |
| LEFT CALF | | |
| RIGHT CALF | | |
| WEIGHT | | |

NOTES

# BODY GOALS

MONTH/YEAR . . . . . . . . . . . .

## THIS MONTH GOALS

## WEEKLY PRIORITIES

*W1*

*W2*

*W3*

*W4*

## OTHER TASKS

## MONTHLY AFFIRMATION

## REVIEW OF THE MONTH

## NOTES

# WATER CHALLENGE

MONTH/YEAR.................

| DAYS | WATER | DAYS | WATER |
| --- | --- | --- | --- |
| 01 | ▽▽▽▽▽▽▽▽ | 16 | ▽▽▽▽▽▽▽▽ |
| 02 | ▽▽▽▽▽▽▽▽ | 17 | ▽▽▽▽▽▽▽▽ |
| 03 | ▽▽▽▽▽▽▽▽ | 18 | ▽▽▽▽▽▽▽▽ |
| 04 | ▽▽▽▽▽▽▽▽ | 19 | ▽▽▽▽▽▽▽▽ |
| 05 | ▽▽▽▽▽▽▽▽ | 20 | ▽▽▽▽▽▽▽▽ |
| 06 | ▽▽▽▽▽▽▽▽ | 21 | ▽▽▽▽▽▽▽▽ |
| 07 | ▽▽▽▽▽▽▽▽ | 22 | ▽▽▽▽▽▽▽▽ |
| 08 | ▽▽▽▽▽▽▽▽ | 23 | ▽▽▽▽▽▽▽▽ |
| 09 | ▽▽▽▽▽▽▽▽ | 24 | ▽▽▽▽▽▽▽▽ |
| 10 | ▽▽▽▽▽▽▽▽ | 25 | ▽▽▽▽▽▽▽▽ |
| 11 | ▽▽▽▽▽▽▽▽ | 26 | ▽▽▽▽▽▽▽▽ |
| 12 | ▽▽▽▽▽▽▽▽ | 27 | ▽▽▽▽▽▽▽▽ |
| 13 | ▽▽▽▽▽▽▽▽ | 28 | ▽▽▽▽▽▽▽▽ |
| 14 | ▽▽▽▽▽▽▽▽ | 29 | ▽▽▽▽▽▽▽▽ |
| 15 | ▽▽▽▽▽▽▽▽ | 30 | ▽▽▽▽▽▽▽▽ |

# BODY PROGRESS TRACKER

## MONTH/YEAR

### WAIST

Week 1: _______________

Week 2: _______________

Week 3: _______________

Week 4: _______________

### ARMS

Week 1: _______________

Week 2: _______________

Week 3: _______________

Week 4: _______________

### THIGHS

Week 1: _______________

Week 2: _______________

Week 3: _______________

Week 4: _______________

### HIPS

Week 1: _______________

Week 2: _______________

Week 3: _______________

Week 4: _______________

| Goal Tracker | Week 1: | Week 2: | Week 3: | Week 4: |
| --- | --- | --- | --- | --- |
| DATE | | | | |
| ARMS | | | | |
| WAIST | | | | |
| HIPS | | | | |
| THIGHS | | | | |
| WEIGHT | | | | |

# BODY MEASUREMENTS TRACKER

## MONTH/YEAR

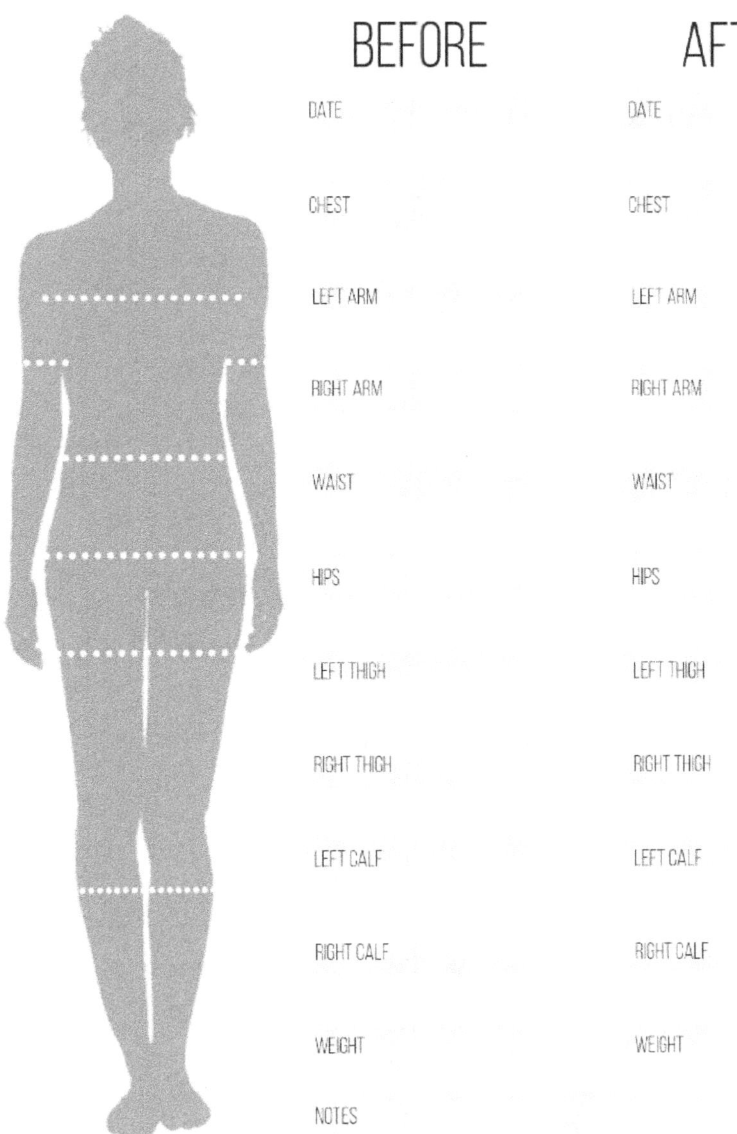

# BODY GOALS

MONTH/YEAR . . . . . . . . . . . .

THIS MONTH
GOALS

WEEKLY
PRIORITIES

W1
W2
W3
W4

OTHER TASKS

MONTHLY
AFFIRMATION

REVIEW OF
THE MONTH

NOTES

# WATER CHALLENGE

MONTH/YEAR.................

| DAYS | WATER | DAYS | WATER |
| --- | --- | --- | --- |
| 01 | ▽▽▽▽▽▽▽▽ | 16 | ▽▽▽▽▽▽▽▽ |
| 02 | ▽▽▽▽▽▽▽▽ | 17 | ▽▽▽▽▽▽▽▽ |
| 03 | ▽▽▽▽▽▽▽▽ | 18 | ▽▽▽▽▽▽▽▽ |
| 04 | ▽▽▽▽▽▽▽▽ | 19 | ▽▽▽▽▽▽▽▽ |
| 05 | ▽▽▽▽▽▽▽▽ | 20 | ▽▽▽▽▽▽▽▽ |
| 06 | ▽▽▽▽▽▽▽▽ | 21 | ▽▽▽▽▽▽▽▽ |
| 07 | ▽▽▽▽▽▽▽▽ | 22 | ▽▽▽▽▽▽▽▽ |
| 08 | ▽▽▽▽▽▽▽▽ | 23 | ▽▽▽▽▽▽▽▽ |
| 09 | ▽▽▽▽▽▽▽▽ | 24 | ▽▽▽▽▽▽▽▽ |
| 10 | ▽▽▽▽▽▽▽▽ | 25 | ▽▽▽▽▽▽▽▽ |
| 11 | ▽▽▽▽▽▽▽▽ | 26 | ▽▽▽▽▽▽▽▽ |
| 12 | ▽▽▽▽▽▽▽▽ | 27 | ▽▽▽▽▽▽▽▽ |
| 13 | ▽▽▽▽▽▽▽▽ | 28 | ▽▽▽▽▽▽▽▽ |
| 14 | ▽▽▽▽▽▽▽▽ | 29 | ▽▽▽▽▽▽▽▽ |
| 15 | ▽▽▽▽▽▽▽▽ | 30 | ▽▽▽▽▽▽▽▽ |

# BODY PROGRESS TRACKER

## MONTH/YEAR

### WAIST

Week 1: _______________

Week 2: _______________

Week 3: _______________

Week 4: _______________

### ARMS

Week 1: _______________

Week 2: _______________

Week 3: _______________

Week 4: _______________

### THIGHS

Week 1: _______________

Week 2: _______________

Week 3: _______________

Week 4: _______________

### HIPS

Week 1: _______________

Week 2: _______________

Week 3: _______________

Week 4: _______________

| Goal Tracker | Week 1: | Week 2: | Week 3: | Week 4: |
|---|---|---|---|---|
| DATE | | | | |
| ARMS | | | | |
| WAIST | | | | |
| HIPS | | | | |
| THIGHS | | | | |
| WEIGHT | | | | |

# BODY MEASUREMENTS TRACKER

## MONTH/YEAR

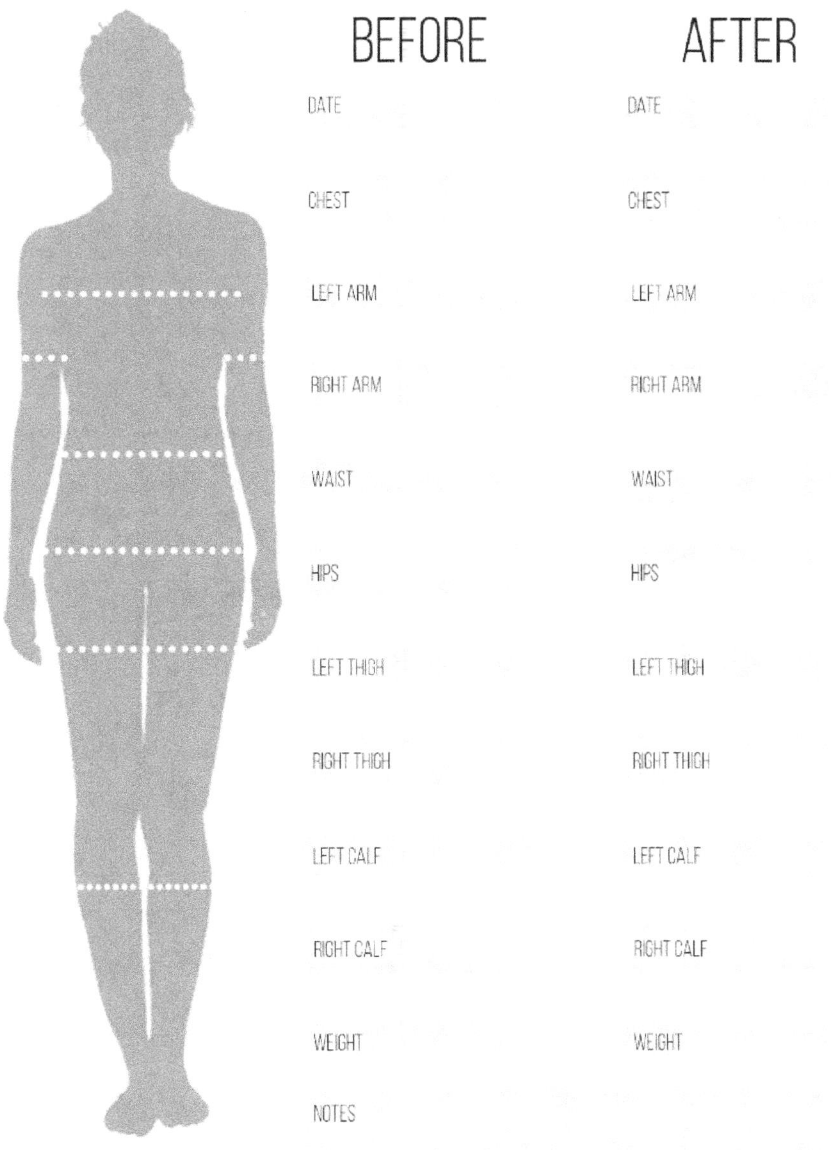

# BODY GOALS

MONTH/YEAR . . . . . . . . . . .

## THIS MONTH GOALS

## WEEKLY PRIORITIES

**W1**
**W2**
**W3**
**W4**

## OTHER TASKS

## MONTHLY AFFIRMATION

## REVIEW OF THE MONTH

## NOTES

# *WATER CHALLENGE*

MONTH/YEAR.................

| DAYS | WATER | DAYS | WATER |
|:----:|:-----:|:----:|:-----:|
| 01 | ▢▢▢▢▢▢▢▢ | 16 | ▢▢▢▢▢▢▢▢ |
| 02 | ▢▢▢▢▢▢▢▢ | 17 | ▢▢▢▢▢▢▢▢ |
| 03 | ▢▢▢▢▢▢▢▢ | 18 | ▢▢▢▢▢▢▢▢ |
| 04 | ▢▢▢▢▢▢▢▢ | 19 | ▢▢▢▢▢▢▢▢ |
| 05 | ▢▢▢▢▢▢▢▢ | 20 | ▢▢▢▢▢▢▢▢ |
| 06 | ▢▢▢▢▢▢▢▢ | 21 | ▢▢▢▢▢▢▢▢ |
| 07 | ▢▢▢▢▢▢▢▢ | 22 | ▢▢▢▢▢▢▢▢ |
| 08 | ▢▢▢▢▢▢▢▢ | 23 | ▢▢▢▢▢▢▢▢ |
| 09 | ▢▢▢▢▢▢▢▢ | 24 | ▢▢▢▢▢▢▢▢ |
| 10 | ▢▢▢▢▢▢▢▢ | 25 | ▢▢▢▢▢▢▢▢ |
| 11 | ▢▢▢▢▢▢▢▢ | 26 | ▢▢▢▢▢▢▢▢ |
| 12 | ▢▢▢▢▢▢▢▢ | 27 | ▢▢▢▢▢▢▢▢ |
| 13 | ▢▢▢▢▢▢▢▢ | 28 | ▢▢▢▢▢▢▢▢ |
| 14 | ▢▢▢▢▢▢▢▢ | 29 | ▢▢▢▢▢▢▢▢ |
| 15 | ▢▢▢▢▢▢▢▢ | 30 | ▢▢▢▢▢▢▢▢ |

# BODY PROGRESS TRACKER
## MONTH/YEAR

### WAIST

Week 1: ___________

Week 2: ___________

Week 3: ___________

Week 4: ___________

### ARMS

Week 1: ___________

Week 2: ___________

Week 3: ___________

Week 4: ___________

### THIGHS

Week 1: ___________

Week 2: ___________

Week 3: ___________

Week 4: ___________

### HIPS

Week 1: ___________

Week 2: ___________

Week 3: ___________

Week 4: ___________

| Goal Tracker | Week 1: | Week 2: | Week 3: | Week 4: |
|---|---|---|---|---|
| DATE | | | | |
| ARMS | | | | |
| WAIST | | | | |
| HIPS | | | | |
| THIGHS | | | | |
| WEIGHT | | | | |

# BODY MEASUREMENTS TRACKER
## MONTH/YEAR

| | BEFORE | AFTER |
|---|---|---|
| DATE | | |
| CHEST | | |
| LEFT ARM | | |
| RIGHT ARM | | |
| WAIST | | |
| HIPS | | |
| LEFT THIGH | | |
| RIGHT THIGH | | |
| LEFT CALF | | |
| RIGHT CALF | | |
| WEIGHT | | |
| NOTES | | |

# BODY GOALS

MONTH/YEAR . . . . . . . . . .

THIS MONTH
GOALS

WEEKLY
PRIORITIES

*W1*
*W2*
*W3*
*W4*

OTHER TASKS

MONTHLY
AFFIRMATION

REVIEW OF
THE MONTH

NOTES

# WATER CHALLENGE

MONTH/YEAR.................

| DAYS | WATER | DAYS | WATER |
|------|-------|------|-------|
| 01 | ▽▽▽▽▽▽▽▽ | 16 | ▽▽▽▽▽▽▽▽ |
| 02 | ▽▽▽▽▽▽▽▽ | 17 | ▽▽▽▽▽▽▽▽ |
| 03 | ▽▽▽▽▽▽▽▽ | 18 | ▽▽▽▽▽▽▽▽ |
| 04 | ▽▽▽▽▽▽▽▽ | 19 | ▽▽▽▽▽▽▽▽ |
| 05 | ▽▽▽▽▽▽▽▽ | 20 | ▽▽▽▽▽▽▽▽ |
| 06 | ▽▽▽▽▽▽▽▽ | 21 | ▽▽▽▽▽▽▽▽ |
| 07 | ▽▽▽▽▽▽▽▽ | 22 | ▽▽▽▽▽▽▽▽ |
| 08 | ▽▽▽▽▽▽▽▽ | 23 | ▽▽▽▽▽▽▽▽ |
| 09 | ▽▽▽▽▽▽▽▽ | 24 | ▽▽▽▽▽▽▽▽ |
| 10 | ▽▽▽▽▽▽▽▽ | 25 | ▽▽▽▽▽▽▽▽ |
| 11 | ▽▽▽▽▽▽▽▽ | 26 | ▽▽▽▽▽▽▽▽ |
| 12 | ▽▽▽▽▽▽▽▽ | 27 | ▽▽▽▽▽▽▽▽ |
| 13 | ▽▽▽▽▽▽▽▽ | 28 | ▽▽▽▽▽▽▽▽ |
| 14 | ▽▽▽▽▽▽▽▽ | 29 | ▽▽▽▽▽▽▽▽ |
| 15 | ▽▽▽▽▽▽▽▽ | 30 | ▽▽▽▽▽▽▽▽ |

# BODY PROGRESS TRACKER
## MONTH/YEAR

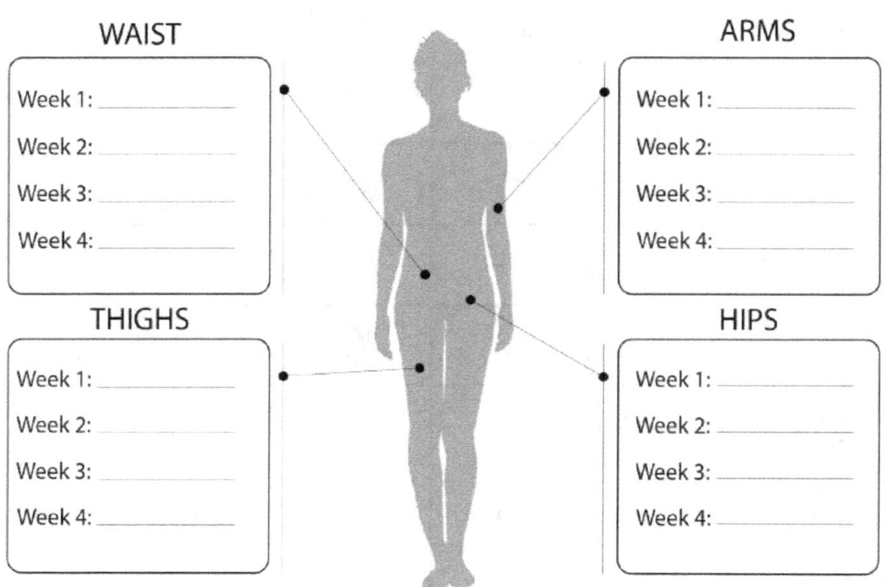



| Goal Tracker | Week 1: | Week 2: | Week 3: | Week 4: |
|---|---|---|---|---|
| DATE | | | | |
| ARMS | | | | |
| WAIST | | | | |
| HIPS | | | | |
| THIGHS | | | | |
| WEIGHT | | | | |

# BODY MEASUREMENTS TRACKER

## MONTH/YEAR

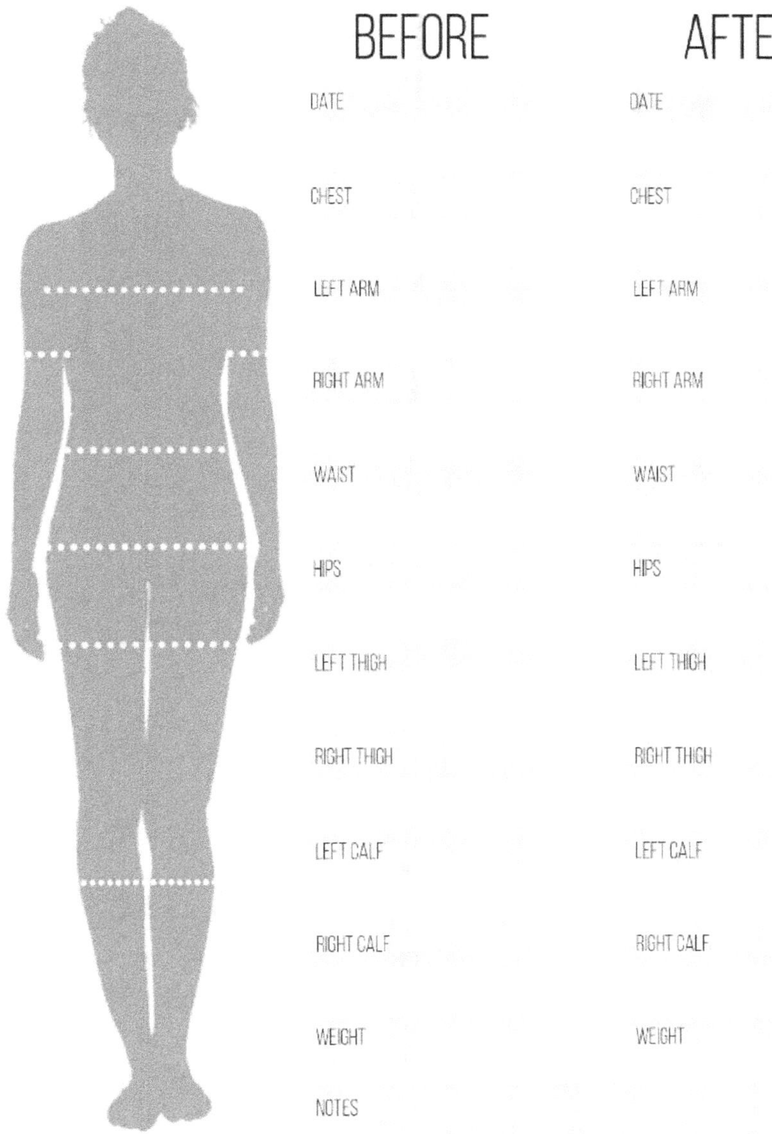

# BODY GOALS

MONTH/YEAR . . . . . . . . . . .

## THIS MONTH GOALS

## WEEKLY PRIORITIES

W1
W2
W3
W4

## OTHER TASKS

## MONTHLY AFFIRMATION

## REVIEW OF THE MONTH

## NOTES

# WATER CHALLENGE

MONTH/YEAR.................

| DAYS | WATER | DAYS | WATER |
|------|-------|------|-------|
| 01 | 🥛🥛🥛🥛🥛🥛🥛🥛 | 16 | 🥛🥛🥛🥛🥛🥛🥛🥛 |
| 02 | 🥛🥛🥛🥛🥛🥛🥛🥛 | 17 | 🥛🥛🥛🥛🥛🥛🥛🥛 |
| 03 | 🥛🥛🥛🥛🥛🥛🥛🥛 | 18 | 🥛🥛🥛🥛🥛🥛🥛🥛 |
| 04 | 🥛🥛🥛🥛🥛🥛🥛🥛 | 19 | 🥛🥛🥛🥛🥛🥛🥛🥛 |
| 05 | 🥛🥛🥛🥛🥛🥛🥛🥛 | 20 | 🥛🥛🥛🥛🥛🥛🥛🥛 |
| 06 | 🥛🥛🥛🥛🥛🥛🥛🥛 | 21 | 🥛🥛🥛🥛🥛🥛🥛🥛 |
| 07 | 🥛🥛🥛🥛🥛🥛🥛🥛 | 22 | 🥛🥛🥛🥛🥛🥛🥛🥛 |
| 08 | 🥛🥛🥛🥛🥛🥛🥛🥛 | 23 | 🥛🥛🥛🥛🥛🥛🥛🥛 |
| 09 | 🥛🥛🥛🥛🥛🥛🥛🥛 | 24 | 🥛🥛🥛🥛🥛🥛🥛🥛 |
| 10 | 🥛🥛🥛🥛🥛🥛🥛🥛 | 25 | 🥛🥛🥛🥛🥛🥛🥛🥛 |
| 11 | 🥛🥛🥛🥛🥛🥛🥛🥛 | 26 | 🥛🥛🥛🥛🥛🥛🥛🥛 |
| 12 | 🥛🥛🥛🥛🥛🥛🥛🥛 | 27 | 🥛🥛🥛🥛🥛🥛🥛🥛 |
| 13 | 🥛🥛🥛🥛🥛🥛🥛🥛 | 28 | 🥛🥛🥛🥛🥛🥛🥛🥛 |
| 14 | 🥛🥛🥛🥛🥛🥛🥛🥛 | 29 | 🥛🥛🥛🥛🥛🥛🥛🥛 |
| 15 | 🥛🥛🥛🥛🥛🥛🥛🥛 | 30 | 🥛🥛🥛🥛🥛🥛🥛🥛 |

# BODY PROGRESS TRACKER

## MONTH/YEAR

### WAIST

Week 1: _______________

Week 2: _______________

Week 3: _______________

Week 4: _______________

### ARMS

Week 1: _______________

Week 2: _______________

Week 3: _______________

Week 4: _______________

### THIGHS

Week 1: _______________

Week 2: _______________

Week 3: _______________

Week 4: _______________

### HIPS

Week 1: _______________

Week 2: _______________

Week 3: _______________

Week 4: _______________

| Goal Tracker | Week 1: | Week 2: | Week 3: | Week 4: |
|---|---|---|---|---|
| DATE | | | | |
| ARMS | | | | |
| WAIST | | | | |
| HIPS | | | | |
| THIGHS | | | | |
| WEIGHT | | | | |

# BODY MEASUREMENTS TRACKER
## MONTH/YEAR

|  | BEFORE | AFTER |
|---|---|---|
| DATE | | |
| CHEST | | |
| LEFT ARM | | |
| RIGHT ARM | | |
| WAIST | | |
| HIPS | | |
| LEFT THIGH | | |
| RIGHT THIGH | | |
| LEFT CALF | | |
| RIGHT CALF | | |
| WEIGHT | | |
| NOTES | | |

# BODY GOALS

MONTH/YEAR . . . . . . . . . .

## THIS MONTH GOALS

## WEEKLY PRIORITIES

*W1*

*W2*

*W3*

*W4*

## OTHER TASKS

## MONTHLY AFFIRMATION

## REVIEW OF THE MONTH

## NOTES

# WATER CHALLENGE

MONTH/YEAR.................

| DAYS | WATER | DAYS | WATER |
|------|-------|------|-------|
| 01 | ▢▢▢▢▢▢▢▢ | 16 | ▢▢▢▢▢▢▢▢ |
| 02 | ▢▢▢▢▢▢▢▢ | 17 | ▢▢▢▢▢▢▢▢ |
| 03 | ▢▢▢▢▢▢▢▢ | 18 | ▢▢▢▢▢▢▢▢ |
| 04 | ▢▢▢▢▢▢▢▢ | 19 | ▢▢▢▢▢▢▢▢ |
| 05 | ▢▢▢▢▢▢▢▢ | 20 | ▢▢▢▢▢▢▢▢ |
| 06 | ▢▢▢▢▢▢▢▢ | 21 | ▢▢▢▢▢▢▢▢ |
| 07 | ▢▢▢▢▢▢▢▢ | 22 | ▢▢▢▢▢▢▢▢ |
| 08 | ▢▢▢▢▢▢▢▢ | 23 | ▢▢▢▢▢▢▢▢ |
| 09 | ▢▢▢▢▢▢▢▢ | 24 | ▢▢▢▢▢▢▢▢ |
| 10 | ▢▢▢▢▢▢▢▢ | 25 | ▢▢▢▢▢▢▢▢ |
| 11 | ▢▢▢▢▢▢▢▢ | 26 | ▢▢▢▢▢▢▢▢ |
| 12 | ▢▢▢▢▢▢▢▢ | 27 | ▢▢▢▢▢▢▢▢ |
| 13 | ▢▢▢▢▢▢▢▢ | 28 | ▢▢▢▢▢▢▢▢ |
| 14 | ▢▢▢▢▢▢▢▢ | 29 | ▢▢▢▢▢▢▢▢ |
| 15 | ▢▢▢▢▢▢▢▢ | 30 | ▢▢▢▢▢▢▢▢ |

# BODY PROGRESS TRACKER

## MONTH/YEAR

### WAIST

Week 1: _______________

Week 2: _______________

Week 3: _______________

Week 4: _______________

### ARMS

Week 1: _______________

Week 2: _______________

Week 3: _______________

Week 4: _______________

### THIGHS

Week 1: _______________

Week 2: _______________

Week 3: _______________

Week 4: _______________

### HIPS

Week 1: _______________

Week 2: _______________

Week 3: _______________

Week 4: _______________

| Goal Tracker | Week 1: | Week 2: | Week 3: | Week 4: |
|---|---|---|---|---|
| DATE | | | | |
| ARMS | | | | |
| WAIST | | | | |
| HIPS | | | | |
| THIGHS | | | | |
| WEIGHT | | | | |

# BODY MEASUREMENTS TRACKER

## MONTH/YEAR

|  | BEFORE | AFTER |
|---|---|---|
| DATE | | DATE |
| CHEST | | CHEST |
| LEFT ARM | | LEFT ARM |
| RIGHT ARM | | RIGHT ARM |
| WAIST | | WAIST |
| HIPS | | HIPS |
| LEFT THIGH | | LEFT THIGH |
| RIGHT THIGH | | RIGHT THIGH |
| LEFT CALF | | LEFT CALF |
| RIGHT CALF | | RIGHT CALF |
| WEIGHT | | WEIGHT |
| NOTES | | |

# BODY GOALS

MONTH/YEAR . . . . . . . . . . .

## THIS MONTH GOALS

## WEEKLY PRIORITIES

W1

W2

W3

W4

## OTHER TASKS

## MONTHLY AFFIRMATION

## REVIEW OF THE MONTH

## NOTES

# *WATER CHALLENGE*

MONTH/YEAR.................

| DAYS | WATER | DAYS | WATER |
|---|---|---|---|
| 01 | ▽▽▽▽▽▽▽▽ | 16 | ▽▽▽▽▽▽▽▽ |
| 02 | ▽▽▽▽▽▽▽▽ | 17 | ▽▽▽▽▽▽▽▽ |
| 03 | ▽▽▽▽▽▽▽▽ | 18 | ▽▽▽▽▽▽▽▽ |
| 04 | ▽▽▽▽▽▽▽▽ | 19 | ▽▽▽▽▽▽▽▽ |
| 05 | ▽▽▽▽▽▽▽▽ | 20 | ▽▽▽▽▽▽▽▽ |
| 06 | ▽▽▽▽▽▽▽▽ | 21 | ▽▽▽▽▽▽▽▽ |
| 07 | ▽▽▽▽▽▽▽▽ | 22 | ▽▽▽▽▽▽▽▽ |
| 08 | ▽▽▽▽▽▽▽▽ | 23 | ▽▽▽▽▽▽▽▽ |
| 09 | ▽▽▽▽▽▽▽▽ | 24 | ▽▽▽▽▽▽▽▽ |
| 10 | ▽▽▽▽▽▽▽▽ | 25 | ▽▽▽▽▽▽▽▽ |
| 11 | ▽▽▽▽▽▽▽▽ | 26 | ▽▽▽▽▽▽▽▽ |
| 12 | ▽▽▽▽▽▽▽▽ | 27 | ▽▽▽▽▽▽▽▽ |
| 13 | ▽▽▽▽▽▽▽▽ | 28 | ▽▽▽▽▽▽▽▽ |
| 14 | ▽▽▽▽▽▽▽▽ | 29 | ▽▽▽▽▽▽▽▽ |
| 15 | ▽▽▽▽▽▽▽▽ | 30 | ▽▽▽▽▽▽▽▽ |

# BODY PROGRESS TRACKER
## MONTH/YEAR

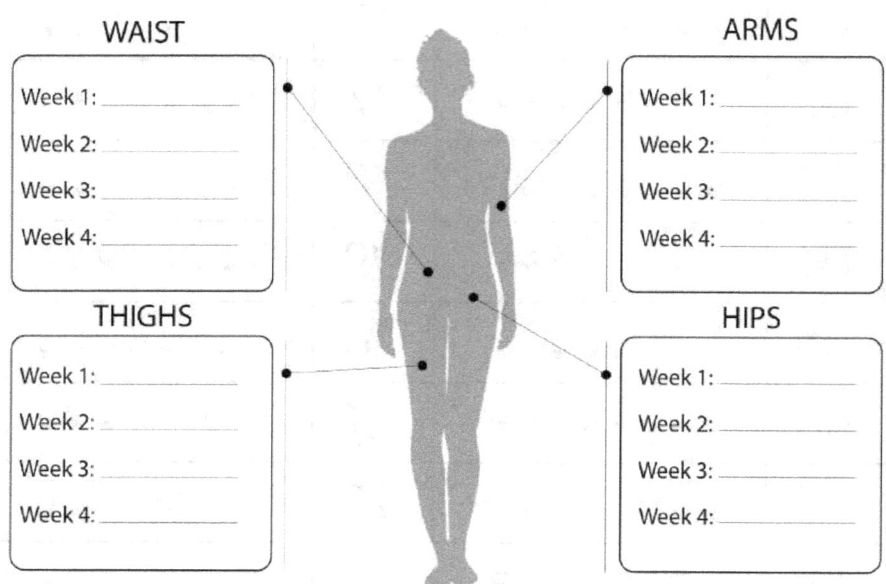

### WAIST

Week 1: _______________

Week 2: _______________

Week 3: _______________

Week 4: _______________

### ARMS

Week 1: _______________

Week 2: _______________

Week 3: _______________

Week 4: _______________

### THIGHS

Week 1: _______________

Week 2: _______________

Week 3: _______________

Week 4: _______________

### HIPS

Week 1: _______________

Week 2: _______________

Week 3: _______________

Week 4: _______________

| Goal Tracker | Week 1: | Week 2: | Week 3: | Week 4: |
|---|---|---|---|---|
| DATE | | | | |
| ARMS | | | | |
| WAIST | | | | |
| HIPS | | | | |
| THIGHS | | | | |
| WEIGHT | | | | |

# BODY MEASUREMENTS TRACKER
## MONTH/YEAR

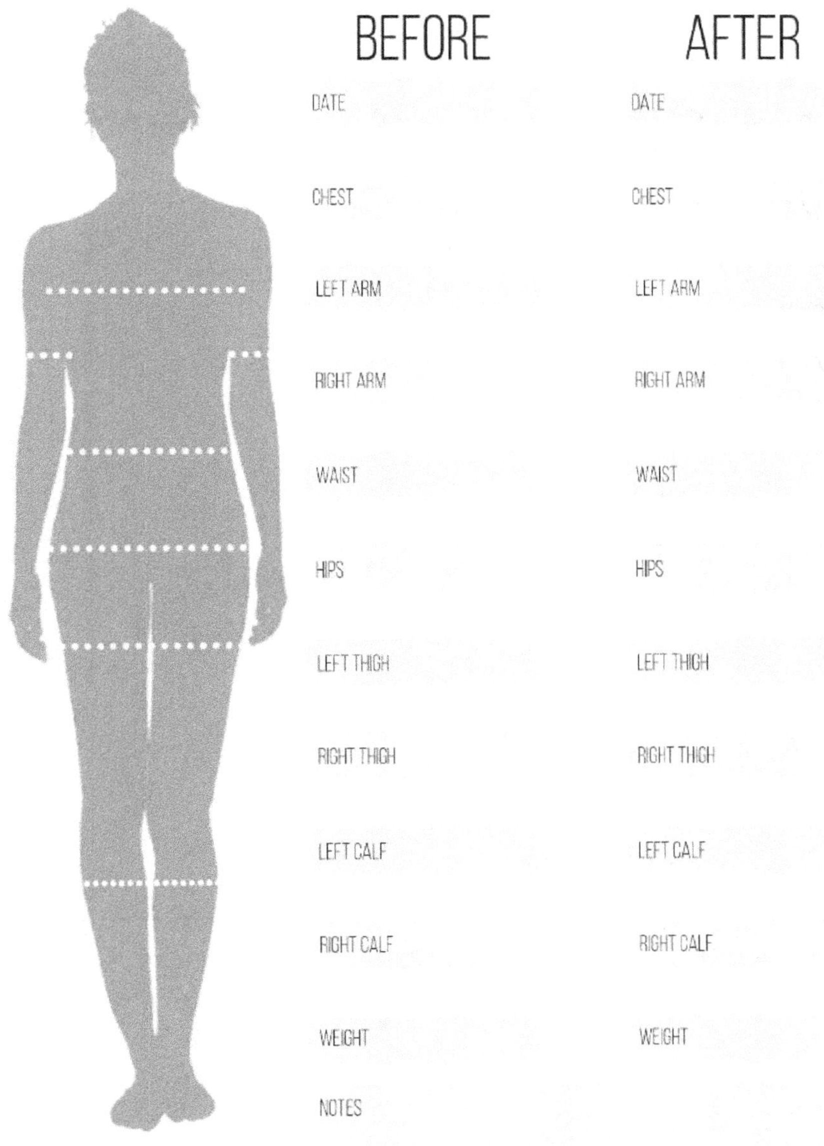

# BODY GOALS

MONTH/YEAR . . . . . . . . . . .

## THIS MONTH
## GOALS

## WEEKLY
## PRIORITIES

W1

W2

W3

W4

## OTHER TASKS

## MONTHLY
## AFFIRMATION

## REVIEW OF
## THE MONTH

## NOTES

# *WATER CHALLENGE*

MONTH/YEAR..................

| DAYS | WATER | DAYS | WATER |
|------|-------|------|-------|
| 01 | ▾▾▾▾▾▾▾▾ | 16 | ▾▾▾▾▾▾▾▾ |
| 02 | ▾▾▾▾▾▾▾▾ | 17 | ▾▾▾▾▾▾▾▾ |
| 03 | ▾▾▾▾▾▾▾▾ | 18 | ▾▾▾▾▾▾▾▾ |
| 04 | ▾▾▾▾▾▾▾▾ | 19 | ▾▾▾▾▾▾▾▾ |
| 05 | ▾▾▾▾▾▾▾▾ | 20 | ▾▾▾▾▾▾▾▾ |
| 06 | ▾▾▾▾▾▾▾▾ | 21 | ▾▾▾▾▾▾▾▾ |
| 07 | ▾▾▾▾▾▾▾▾ | 22 | ▾▾▾▾▾▾▾▾ |
| 08 | ▾▾▾▾▾▾▾▾ | 23 | ▾▾▾▾▾▾▾▾ |
| 09 | ▾▾▾▾▾▾▾▾ | 24 | ▾▾▾▾▾▾▾▾ |
| 10 | ▾▾▾▾▾▾▾▾ | 25 | ▾▾▾▾▾▾▾▾ |
| 11 | ▾▾▾▾▾▾▾▾ | 26 | ▾▾▾▾▾▾▾▾ |
| 12 | ▾▾▾▾▾▾▾▾ | 27 | ▾▾▾▾▾▾▾▾ |
| 13 | ▾▾▾▾▾▾▾▾ | 28 | ▾▾▾▾▾▾▾▾ |
| 14 | ▾▾▾▾▾▾▾▾ | 29 | ▾▾▾▾▾▾▾▾ |
| 15 | ▾▾▾▾▾▾▾▾ | 30 | ▾▾▾▾▾▾▾▾ |

# BODY PROGRESS TRACKER

## MONTH/YEAR ................

### WAIST

Week 1: _____________

Week 2: _____________

Week 3: _____________

Week 4: _____________

### ARMS

Week 1: _____________

Week 2: _____________

Week 3: _____________

Week 4: _____________

### THIGHS

Week 1: _____________

Week 2: _____________

Week 3: _____________

Week 4: _____________

### HIPS

Week 1: _____________

Week 2: _____________

Week 3: _____________

Week 4: _____________

| Goal Tracker | Week 1: | Week 2: | Week 3: | Week 4: |
|---|---|---|---|---|
| DATE | | | | |
| ARMS | | | | |
| WAIST | | | | |
| HIPS | | | | |
| THIGHS | | | | |
| WEIGHT | | | | |

# BODY MEASUREMENTS TRACKER

## MONTH/YEAR

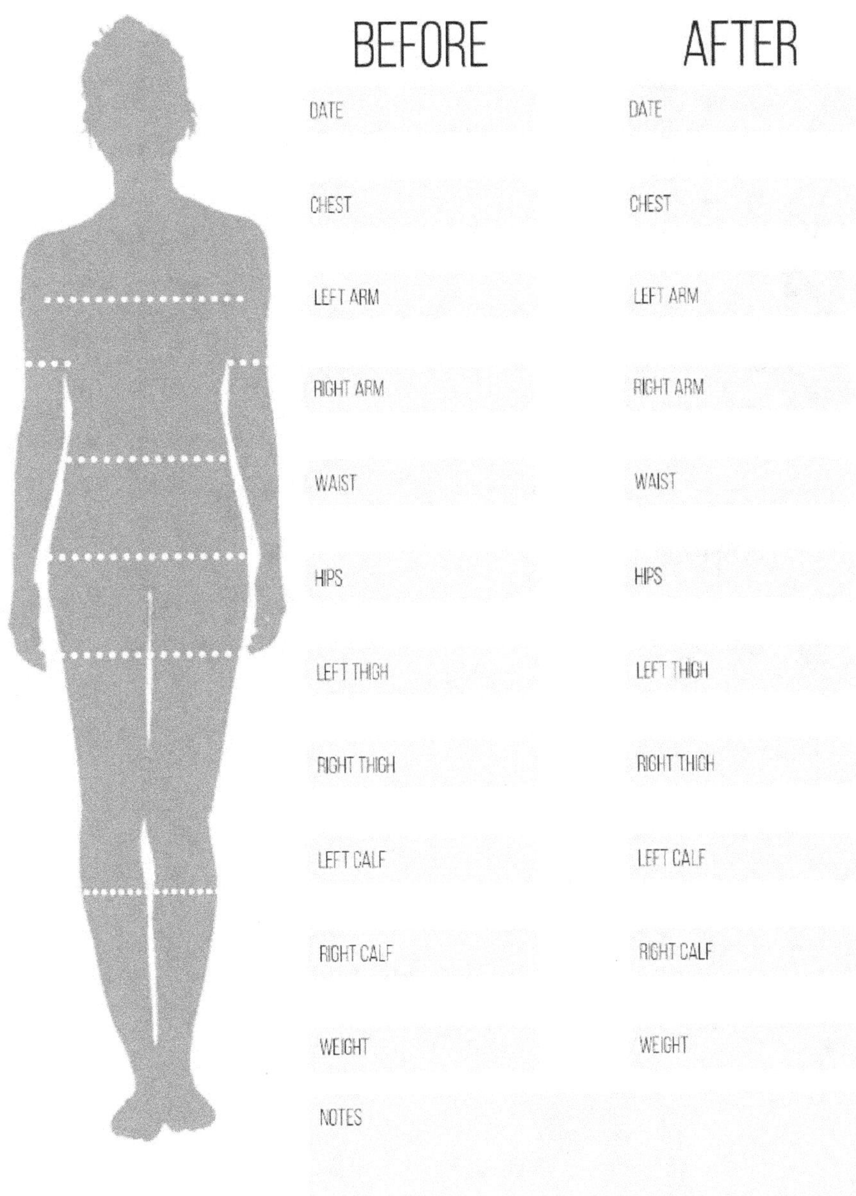

# BODY GOALS

MONTH/YEAR . . . . . . . . . .

THIS MONTH
GOALS

WEEKLY
PRIORITIES

W1
W2
W3
W4

OTHER TASKS

MONTHLY
AFFIRMATION

REVIEW OF
THE MONTH

NOTES

# WATER CHALLENGE

MONTH/YEAR.................

| DAYS | WATER | DAYS | WATER |
|------|-------|------|-------|
| 01 | 🥛🥛🥛🥛🥛🥛🥛🥛 | 16 | 🥛🥛🥛🥛🥛🥛🥛🥛 |
| 02 | 🥛🥛🥛🥛🥛🥛🥛🥛 | 17 | 🥛🥛🥛🥛🥛🥛🥛🥛 |
| 03 | 🥛🥛🥛🥛🥛🥛🥛🥛 | 18 | 🥛🥛🥛🥛🥛🥛🥛🥛 |
| 04 | 🥛🥛🥛🥛🥛🥛🥛🥛 | 19 | 🥛🥛🥛🥛🥛🥛🥛🥛 |
| 05 | 🥛🥛🥛🥛🥛🥛🥛🥛 | 20 | 🥛🥛🥛🥛🥛🥛🥛🥛 |
| 06 | 🥛🥛🥛🥛🥛🥛🥛🥛 | 21 | 🥛🥛🥛🥛🥛🥛🥛🥛 |
| 07 | 🥛🥛🥛🥛🥛🥛🥛🥛 | 22 | 🥛🥛🥛🥛🥛🥛🥛🥛 |
| 08 | 🥛🥛🥛🥛🥛🥛🥛🥛 | 23 | 🥛🥛🥛🥛🥛🥛🥛🥛 |
| 09 | 🥛🥛🥛🥛🥛🥛🥛🥛 | 24 | 🥛🥛🥛🥛🥛🥛🥛🥛 |
| 10 | 🥛🥛🥛🥛🥛🥛🥛🥛 | 25 | 🥛🥛🥛🥛🥛🥛🥛🥛 |
| 11 | 🥛🥛🥛🥛🥛🥛🥛🥛 | 26 | 🥛🥛🥛🥛🥛🥛🥛🥛 |
| 12 | 🥛🥛🥛🥛🥛🥛🥛🥛 | 27 | 🥛🥛🥛🥛🥛🥛🥛🥛 |
| 13 | 🥛🥛🥛🥛🥛🥛🥛🥛 | 28 | 🥛🥛🥛🥛🥛🥛🥛🥛 |
| 14 | 🥛🥛🥛🥛🥛🥛🥛🥛 | 29 | 🥛🥛🥛🥛🥛🥛🥛🥛 |
| 15 | 🥛🥛🥛🥛🥛🥛🥛🥛 | 30 | 🥛🥛🥛🥛🥛🥛🥛🥛 |